Collins

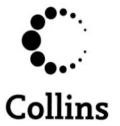

need to know?

Detox

Gill Paul

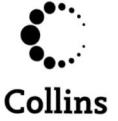

Collins

First published in 2007 by Collins
an imprint of
HarperCollins Publishers
77–85 Fulham Palace Road
London W6 8JB

www.collins.co.uk

Collins is a registered trademark of HarperCollins Publishers Limited

10 09 08 07
7 6 5 4 3 2 1

© HarperCollins Publishers, 2007

All rights reserved. No part of this publication may be reproduced, stored in a retrieval system, or transmitted, in any form or by any means, electronic, mechanical, photocopying, recording or otherwise, without the prior written permission of the publishers.

A catalogue record for this book is available from the British Library

Text: Gill Paul
Recipes: Kate Santon
Editor: Heather Thomas
Designer: Rolando Ugolini
Series design: Mark Thomson
Front cover photograph: Emely/zefa/Corbis
Back cover photographs: Getty Images
Photography: Getty Images

ISBN-13: 978-00-0720224-9
ISBN-10: 0-00-720224-5

Printed and bound by Printing Express Ltd, Hong Kong

Important
This is a general reference book and although care has been taken to ensure the information is as up-to-date and accurate as possible, it is no substitute for professional advice based on your personal circumstances. Consult your doctor before making any major changes to your diet or activity levels or before taking any over-the-counter medicines, especially if you have any pre-existing health problems. Information on specific dieting methods is provided for reference and should not be taken as a recommendation or endorsement.

Contents

1 **How toxic are you?** 6
2 **How detoxing works** 32
3 **What to eat and drink** 56
4 **Detox recipes** 80
5 **Detox aids** 114
6 **Holistic detox therapies** 132
7 **Toxins that surround us** 150
8 **Emotional detoxing** 170

Glossary 188
Need to know more? 189
Index 191

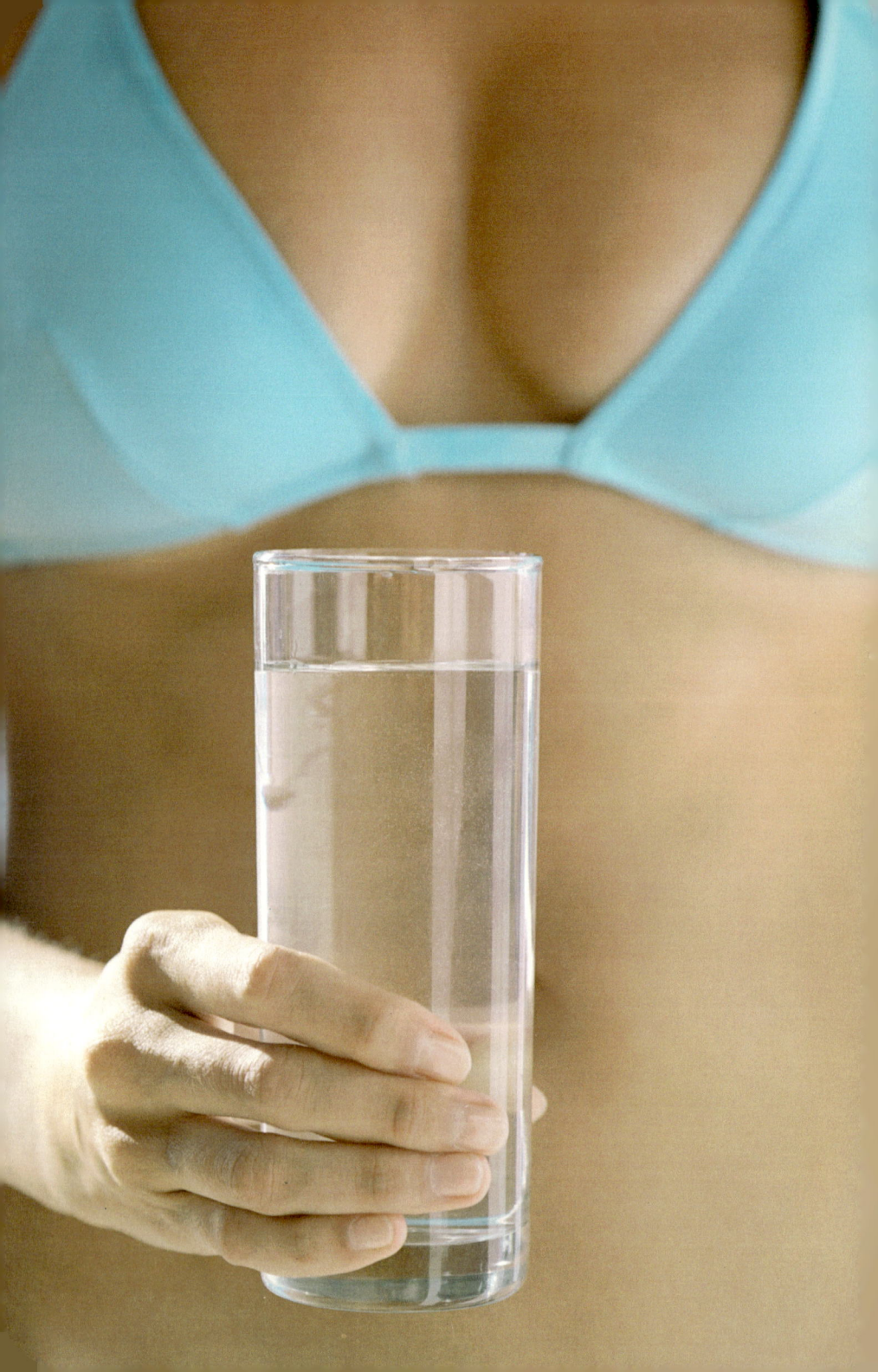

1 How toxic are you?

The human body is extremely sophisticated, performing a huge range of essential functions simultaneously right round the clock. Among these functions is the crucial one of filtering out and eliminating any materials that could cause the body harm. Over the centuries, as technology has developed, the toxins to which humans are exposed have changed and the body has adapted to deal with new ones, but in the last 60 years there has been a massive increase in the number of chemicals in our air, water, food and everyday surroundings. Are we still coping? Or are we heading for overload?

1 How toxic are you?

Your body's defences

The liver, kidneys, spleen, digestive system, respiratory system, lymphatic system and skin all work together to try and keep potentially harmful substances (toxins) out of our bodies, or to neutralize them if they do get in. So how well are your body's defences working?

must know

Smoking
Cigarettes contain up to 600 additives and when these are set on fire, the smoke contains over 4,000 chemicals, of which over 50 are known to be cancer-forming. They include radioactive Polonium-210, found in tobacco that is grown in fields which are fertilized with phosphates, and Zyklon B, a gas that was used by the Nazis for mass extermination in the death camps.

What is a toxin?

Toxins are substances that can harm us when they are ingested into the body. If asked to name some toxins, most people would mention alcohol, tobacco and caffeine first, and they would be right in so far as these are all substances that can cause significant harm to the body. They are deliberately ingested toxins, but there are many more that we don't consume deliberately and may not even be aware of. Some are in the air we breathe, the water we drink and the foods, even seemingly healthy ones, that we eat.

When you eat a strawberry that has been sprayed with pesticide to kill any bugs in the strawberry patch, you ingest the pesticide along with the vitamin C and antioxidants of the fruit. When you stand on a city street and breathe in, your lungs have to cope with a cocktail of exhaust fumes and other gases, among which is the oxygen we need to stay alive. When you drink mineral water, you could be consuming traces of antimony, a poison that has been found in plastic bottles, alongside the water we need for survival.

We are surrounded by toxins at every turn, no matter how hard we try to be healthy. Fortunately, however, our bodies have ways of dealing with most of the substances they come into contact with.

Prevention is the best defence
To get into the body, toxins have to be inhaled, eaten or absorbed through the skin. The first-line defences try to prevent entry in the first place but, if they fail, there are second and third lines in waiting.

Respiratory system
When you breathe in through your nose, some tiny hairs – cilia – filter out particles of dust and soot, which will be expelled the next time you sneeze or blow your nose. The mucous membranes lining the mouth and nose contain a chemical called lactoferrin, which destroys bacteria, and saliva also has a host of antibacterial ingredients. As air travels down the respiratory tract, more cilia and mucous membranes remove any unwanted particles and phlegm is produced to ferry them upwards, triggering sensors that induce us to cough.

Once in the lungs, the air enters sacs known as alveoli, and there the white blood cells identify any dust or potential toxins that have made it through the other defences and they release the appropriate toxin-killing cells. At least, this is the case in normal, healthy adults; those with asthma or other lung problems don't fight toxins quite so successfully.

Digestive system
When you eat or drink something, the antibacterial compounds in the mouth work on it first, and then stomach acid kills off a lot of potentially dangerous toxins before they get further down the intestine.

> **must know**
>
> **A good weep**
> The eyes have their own defence system to prevent toxins getting in. Our eyelashes sweep away larger particles, while our tears contain an enzyme called lysozyme, which can destroy bacteria, and the liquid washes away micro-organisms.

1 How toxic are you?

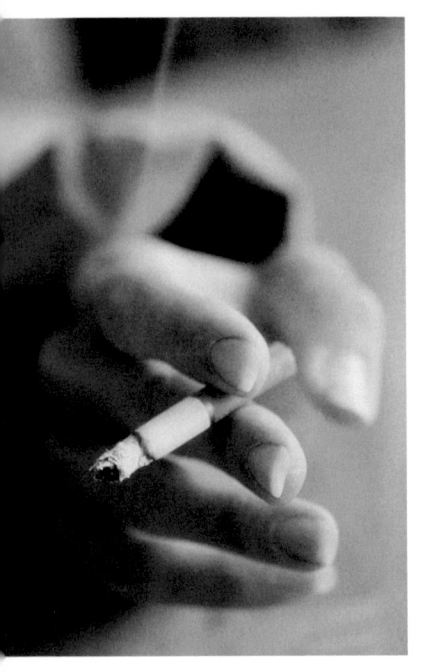

Once in the intestine, beneficial bacteria (known as 'friendly' in the TV ads) help to defend the system from poisons while microscopic villi – little fingers which are lined with capillaries – absorb nutrients into the blood stream. The small intestine, which is 6m (20ft) in length, filters out any larger molecules and undigested foods and carries them down to be excreted when you have a bowel movement. Smaller molecules that are absorbed are carried in the first instance to the liver.

Liver and gall bladder

The liver is a multi-tasking organ which produces and processes hundreds of chemicals every day. When blood arrives from the small intestine, the liver secretes enzymes that process vital nutrients into a form in which they can be used by the cells of the body. It stores excess glucose (sugar) as glycogen and produces cholesterol, a substance that helps the blood to carry fats around the body. It also clears the blood of drugs and poisons, breaking them down to neutralize them or turning them into a form in which they can be secreted as bile fluid.

Bile is transported from the liver to the gall bladder. When you next eat something containing fat, the bile is excreted into the small intestine to help the digestive process and, if the system is functioning effectively, the bile will then pass from your body in faeces.

Kidneys

The kidneys filter about 200 litres of blood every day, sifting out waste products and excess water. A series of tiny tubes called nephrons are the

Everyone knows that smoking causes lung damage, but not so many are aware that it also harms the stomach lining, liver, kidneys, blood vessels and heart.

filtering units. Most of us will form about 2 litres (3½ pints) of urine a day from substances that are no longer needed by the body.

Spleen
Another of the body's filtering systems, the spleen removes worn-out red blood cells from circulation and recycles them into iron to build the blood. It also gets rid of any unhealthy bacteria, so it can stop you going down with colds or flu when it is functioning efficiently.

Lymphatic system
White blood cells (the ones that fight disease) are stored in lymph nodes situated under your arms, in your neck, around your spine and in your groin. You may be able to feel that your lymph nodes are swollen when you are fighting off an infection. A watery fluid called lymph is circulated round the body, mainly by the action of your muscles. The lymphatic system does not have a pump – in the way that the blood circulates due to the action of the heart – so it can be sluggish if you don't get much exercise.

In the cells, lymph is responsible for filtering out the waste products of cellular reactions and other toxins that have got into the tissues. It also carries white blood cells to sites of infection, where they adhere to and break down micro-organisms and debris that they recognize as foreign.

Skin
The average adult has 1.6 square metres (3 square yards) of skin forming a barrier between the body's

> **must know**
>
> **Bowel movements**
> Ideally, food remains should pass through the digestive system within 24 hours. However, most British adults retain waste products in their colon for between two and seven days – in some cases, much longer – meaning that toxic substances have a good chance of being reabsorbed into the bloodstream again.

1 How toxic are you?

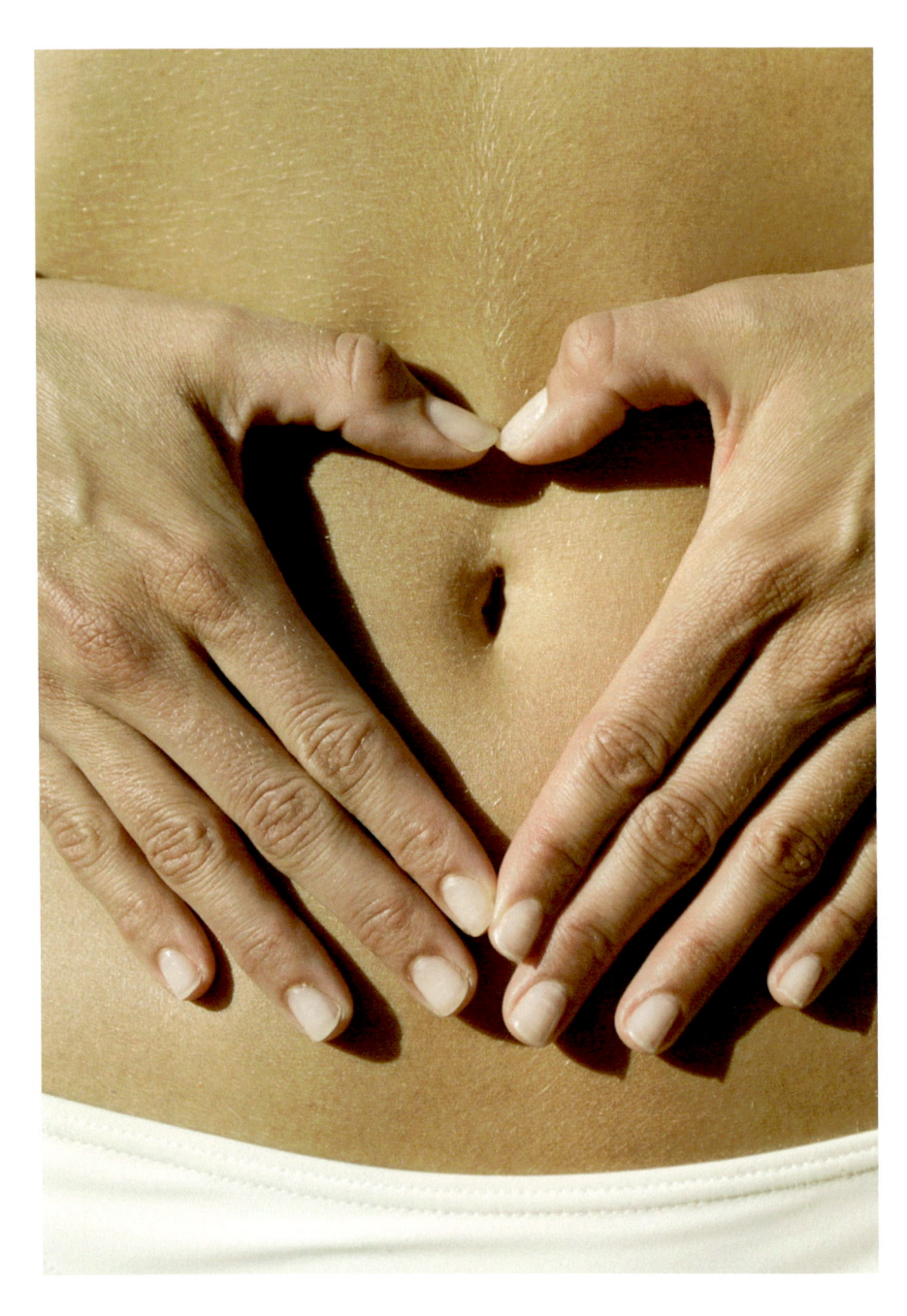

internal organs and the outside world. Bacteria and micro-organisms cannot pass through unbroken skin, and they are prevented from multiplying by the action of oily sebum secreted by the sebaceous glands at the root of hair follicles. Sweat also contains antibacterial lactoferrin. However, if the skin is broken, by a cut or graze, bacteria and micro-organisms can get into the body and the immune system has to send white blood cells to kill them. Chemicals are released that cause the area to become red, hot and inflamed as blood vessels widen to speed white blood cells to the site.

Some chemicals can pass through unbroken skin, but only very slowly. Thus the nicotine in nicotine patches makes its way into the bloodstream, and so do certain toxic chemicals, such as insecticides and solvents, which can cause problems.

The skin is also an organ for the secretion of waste products. As you heat up and perspire, you release a mixture of urea along with other toxins from the fatty tissues. The more you sweat, the more you release, which is why saunas can be an effective part of a general detox programme.

Overload of waste disposal systems

With so many front-line defences and back-up systems, it is hard to see how any unwanted invaders still break through into our internal tissues and organs. But a number of research organizations have carried out sophisticated tests on generally healthy members of the public and found that they are loaded with huge quantities of toxic chemicals.

In 1999 and 2000, the American Centers for Disease Control and Prevention tested 2,500 people

Opposite: Detoxing can help your gut work much more efficiently and helps to prevent bloating.

> **must know**
>
> **Hormone trouble**
> Toxins in the blood disturb the action of our hormones, leading to problems, such as acne in teenagers, PMS (premenstrual syndrome), heavy periods and menopausal symptoms in women, and hair loss in men. Conventional medical treatments for these problems often involve taking synthetic hormones, such as the Pill or HRT (hormone replacement therapy), which just add another layer of circulating hormones for the liver to deal with.

1 How toxic are you?

must know

Autism

In his 2006 book *Autism, Brain and Environment*, Richard Lathe suggests that the huge increase in cases of autism in recent years could be due to an increase in environmental toxins, including pesticides, lead, PCBs and mercury. He suggests that many cases are caused by a genetic weakness that means the system can't deal adequately with such toxins, leading to brain damage that causes the psychological problems connected with the syndrome.

for 116 different toxic chemicals and found that in every single case, they were storing several of them. *The Sunday Times* published similar findings in the UK in 2004. In all instances, they were able to measure scary levels of toxic chemicals in the volunteers' blood and tissues, including the following: polychlorinated biphenyls (PCBs), which have been banned since the 1970s; DDT, a pesticide banned in the UK and US; dioxins; and heavy metals, including lead, cadmium, mercury and aluminium. The problem is that so many new chemicals have been launched over the last 60 years that the body's defences have not had time to adapt or find ways of fighting them off.

Did you know?

• More than 80,000 different industrial chemicals are now licensed for use.
• The average British adult is thought to consume 5kg (11lb) of food additives a year, and 4.5 litres (8 pints) of pesticides on their fruit and vegetables.
• Up to 25 per cent of the US population suffer from heavy metal poisoning from lead, cadmium, mercury and aluminium. Heavy metal toxicity is linked to several diseases, including Alzheimer's, Parkinson's and certain severe neurological conditions.
• In 1940, it took four months to raise a chicken from when it hatched until it weighed around 2kg (4lb) and was ready to eat. In 1990, it took just six weeks because the additives in chicken food have been designed to fatten them up quickly. These same additives can make it harder for us to lose weight when we have ingested them through

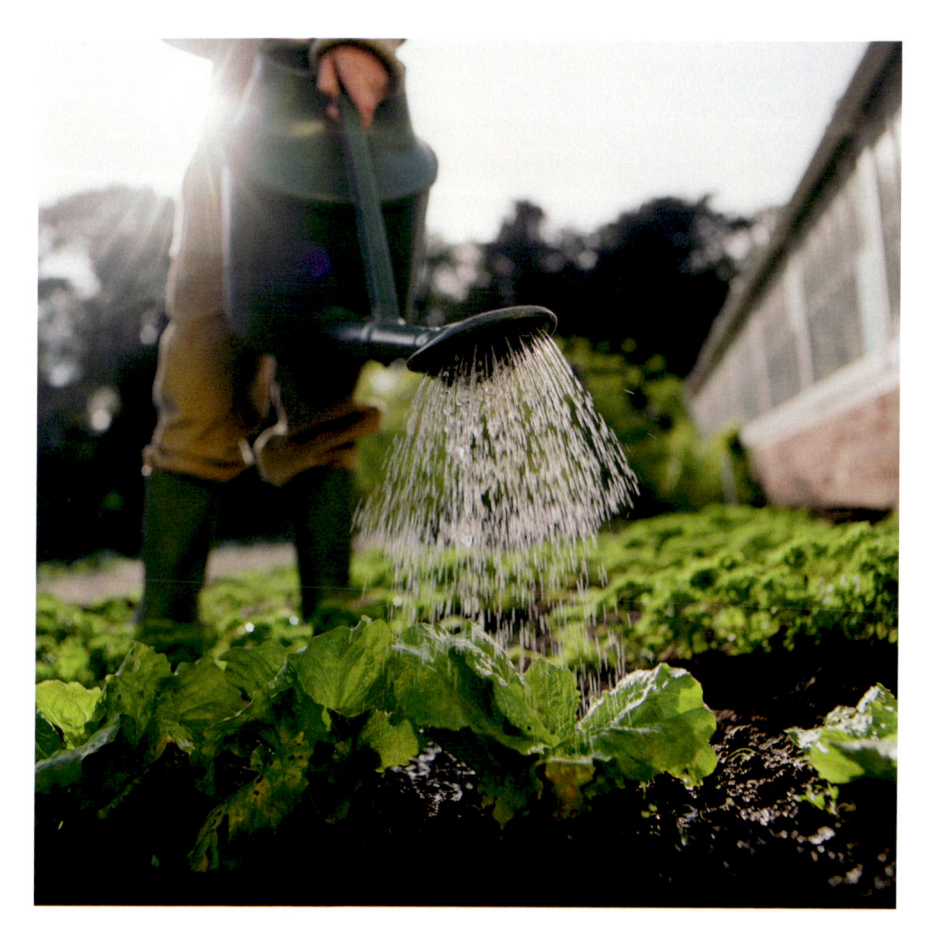

eating chicken. Battery-farm-reared chickens are also chock-full of antibiotics, which are given to them routinely to prevent disease in their overcrowded conditions.

- More and more fish caught around the world contain such high levels of mercury that national governments are advising pregnant women not to eat the larger fish, such as tuna, which have the highest concentrations. One study found that women who ate more than two servings of fish per

Explore non-toxic methods of pest management if you grow your own vegetables and fruit.

1 How toxic are you?

must know

Heavy metals
Arsenic, cadmium, lead and mercury cannot be broken down in the body so they accumulate and cause damage at even low levels. They are found in all sorts of common substances:
• Arsenic can be ingested from food and water that has been contaminated, or from breathing smoke from burning wood that has been treated with copper-chromated arsenic.
• Cadmium can be found in water and foods that come from the water, especially shellfish.
• Lead is found in pipes, paints and solder in old houses.
• Mercury is found in dental fillings, vaccinations, and contaminated fish and shellfish.

The water supplies in many areas can contain nitrate levels above specified EU limits, soaked up from fertilizers in the soil.

week had a higher risk of having a child with autism; 57 per cent of mothers of children with attention deficit disorder were found to have high levels of mercury in their bodies.
• Fluoride, added to tap water in many areas to protect the teeth, can build up in the soil, in plants and in our bones. It can cause osteoporosis, and some studies link it to hypothyroidism, which affects 10–25 per cent of the British population. Fluoride can make it harder for the immune system to distinguish foreign substances from the body's own tissue, leading to skin rashes and intestinal disorders, while several studies link fluoride with genetic disorders.
• Chemicals that mimic the effects of oestrogen in the body are present in a wide range of household cleaning products, including some washing-up liquids and fabric softeners – and cosmetics, such as lipstick and nail polish, as well as hair dyes and many other substances found in the average home. This is one cause of oestrogen dominance, a hormonal imbalance that affects men and women throughout the Western world.
• Formaldehyde, found in new carpets and processed wood furniture among other things, can irritate the eyes, nose and throat at just low levels.
• A ready-washed bag of salad contains chlorine levels 20 times higher than in most swimming pools. Chlorine was one of the poisonous gases used to kill the enemy in World War I.
• Volatile organic compounds (VOCs) are found in aerosol sprays, dry-cleaned clothing, paint, paint strippers and petrol – in fact, there are more than 200 VOCs in common UK household products.

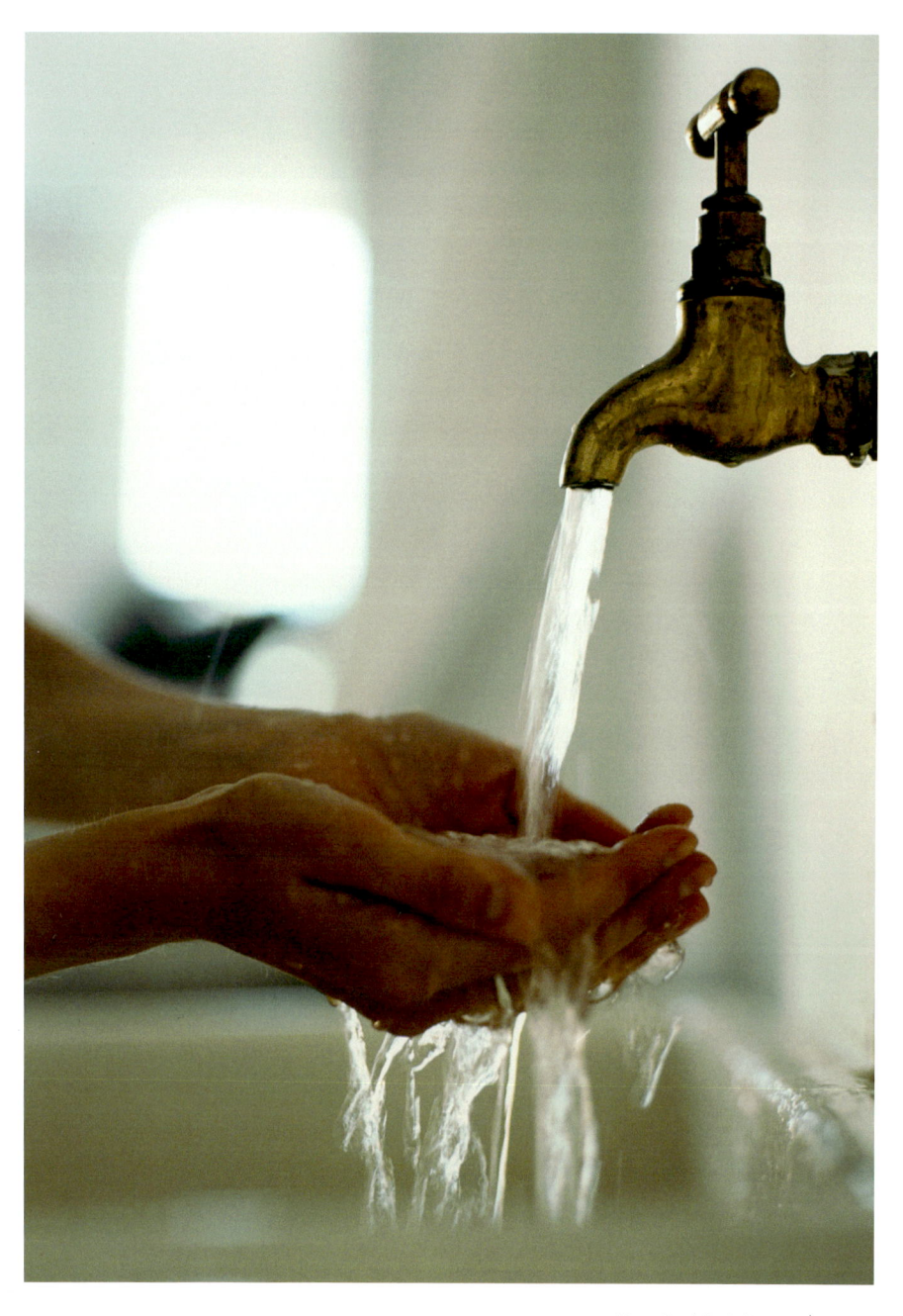

1 How toxic are you?

Food additives

Long lists of E numbers in the ingredients of a foodstuff should make you wary. Some have protective or preservative functions, but others are just used to colour foods or enhance flavours. The following have all been associated with the side effects noted:

- Tartrazine (E102) – may suppress the immune system and can cause hyperactivity in children, allergies, asthma, migraines, even cancer.
- Sunset yellow (E110) – can be particularly dangerous for asthmatics and for anyone who is sensitive to aspirin.
- Amaranth (E123) – may suppress the immune system and has been banned in the US since 1976.
- Erythrosine (E127) – mimics the action of oestrogen in the body and can be carcinogenic.
- Sodium benzoate (E211) – linked to behaviour problems in children.
- Calcium propionate (E282) – linked to attention deficit and sleep problems in children.
- Butylated hydroxyanisole (BTGA – E320) – linked to attention deficit, irritability and asthma; banned in Japan.
- Monosodium glutamate (E621) – can cause headaches, giddiness, nausea, muscle pains, heart palpitations, irritability, attention problems.
- Ribonucleotides (E635) – linked to allergies and behaviour problems in children.
- Aspartame (E951) – linked to headaches, mood swings, fatigue and allergies.

Note: This list could stretch over several pages – in fact, there are many entire books about the huge quantities of brand-new toxins that are being created by industry, and plenty of evidence that these toxins are making their way through our bodies' defence systems to be stored in the fatty tissue, blood and bones.

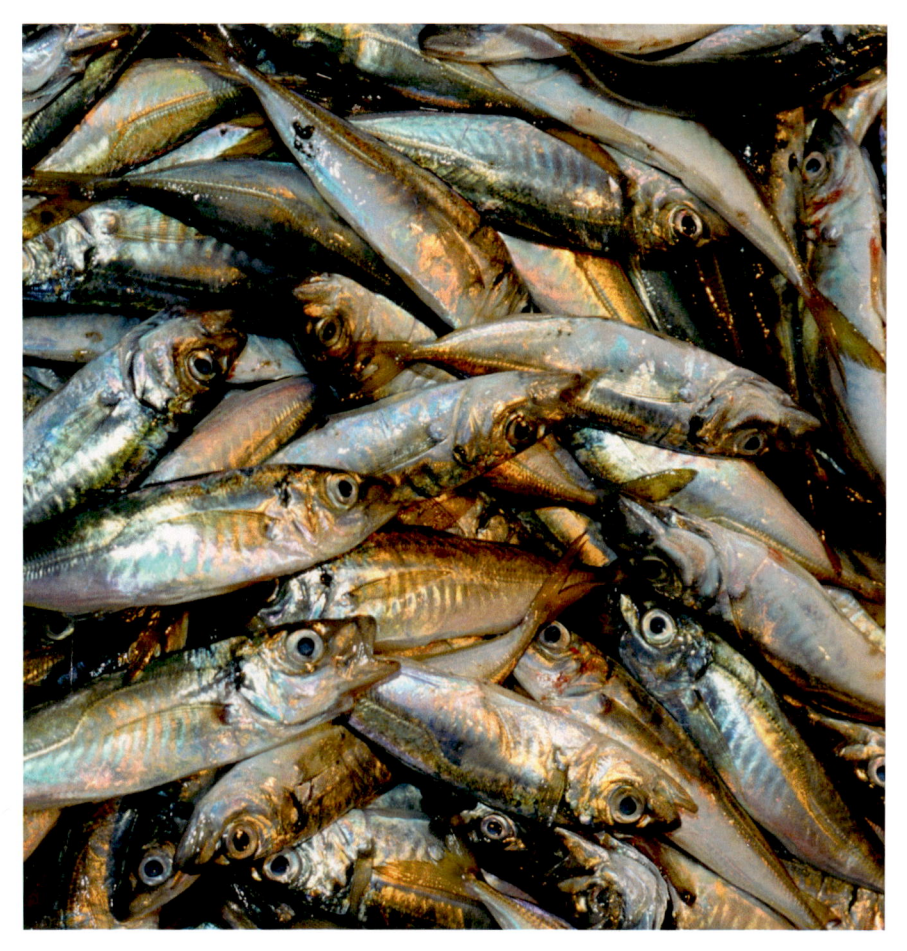

Some studies indicate that VOCs may damage the nervous and immune systems and that they have been linked to brain tumours, childhood leukaemia and childhood asthma.

• Phthalates, which are used to make all sorts of household goods from toys to wallpaper, have been linked to liver and thyroid damage, cancer, low sperm counts in men, miscarriages in women, and birth defects in babies.

We are advised to eat oily fish twice a week for the essential fatty acids they contain, but it may be best to avoid big fish such as tuna and swordfish.

1 How toxic are you?

What toxins do to us

We have looked at how the body's waste disposal systems work in 'normal' circumstances, but what can go wrong if they become overloaded with more toxins than they can deal with, or with new ones that they do not recognize?

must know

Stress
When we are stressed, our heartbeat rises, more sugar is released into the bloodstream and the hormones cortisol and adrenaline are released, both of which promote fat storage in the abdomen. People who are frequently stressed are prone to getting into a pattern of compulsive eating, drinking or smoking. Stress is a toxic emotion all round. See Chapter 8 for ways of combatting it.

Underfunctioning lungs

When they are assaulted daily by air pollutants, the cilia and the mucous membranes in the respiratory system become less effective. The alveoli get furred up with tarry substances, meaning that less of the surface area across which oxygen is absorbed to the blood is available. Less oxygen in the system makes us get tired more easily, so our muscles ache more readily on exertion. Overall, we feel more sluggish.

The incidence of asthma has been rising steadily since 1970. It is now four times higher in adults and six times higher in children than it was back then. According to Asthma UK, environmental pollution may play a part in causing it and certainly makes symptoms worse. The weight of medical evidence suggests that active or passive exposure to cigarette smoke in the early years of life increases the risk of developing asthma.

About 15 per cent of the population in industrialized countries now suffer from hay fever. It has a much higher prevalence in urban areas than rural settings, and increases are particularly striking in areas of high pollution. Like asthma, it is an allergic disease, but it seems that our atmosphere is making us much more prone to these conditions, and, once you have a respiratory disease like this, it becomes harder for your lungs to fight off other toxins.

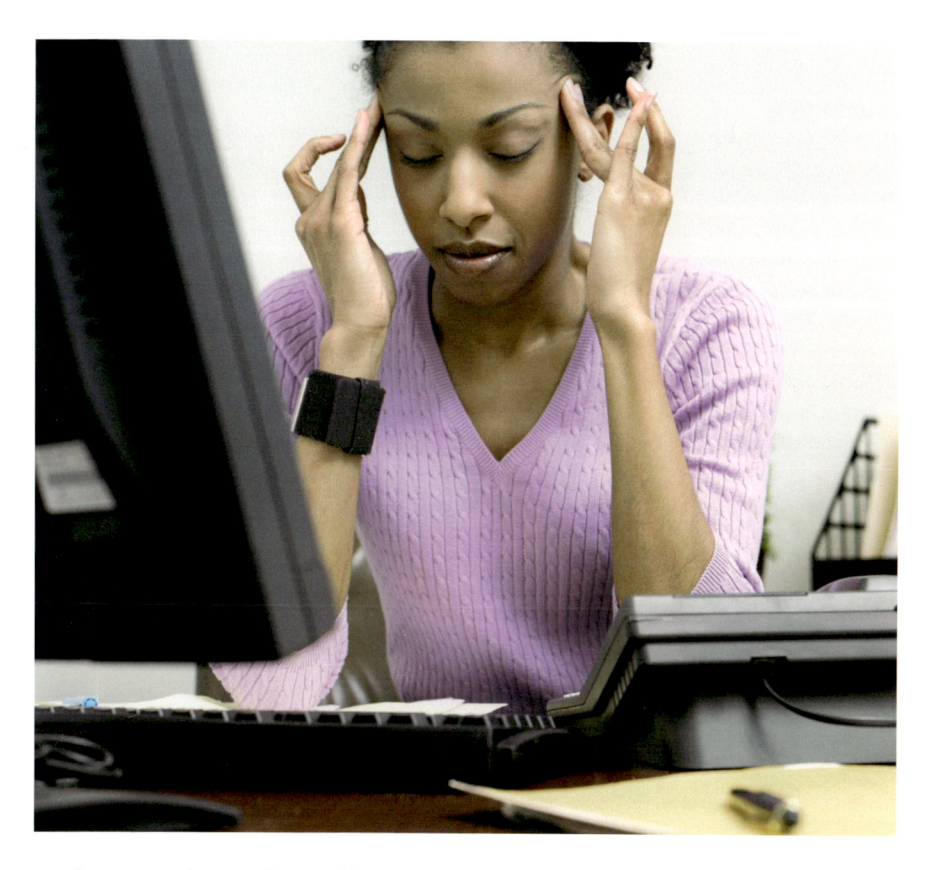

Leaky gut
Only a few substances are absorbed directly through the stomach, and these include alcohol, aspirin, cigarette smoke and certain other noxious chemicals. If the stomach lining has been assaulted too often in this way, it can become 'leaky'. Further down in the intestine, the same thing can happen due to our intake of antibiotics, caffeine, chemicals in processed foods, prescription corticosteroids, or even just a diet

A mild headache in your temples after eating a fatty meal means that your liver is sluggish.

1 How toxic are you?

> **must know**
>
> **Coeliac disease**
> This is a hypersensitivity to gluten, a protein that is found in wheat and rye and certain other cereals. The damage it causes to the gut can prevent absorption of other foods, leading to vitamin and mineral deficiencies, weight loss, abdominal pain, tiredness and a host of other unpleasant symptoms. Once the sensitivity develops, it is permanent, and the only thing you can do is to avoid gluten for the rest of your life.

that is full of highly refined carbohydrates, such as sweets, cakes, biscuits, white bread and pizza.

Once you have a 'leaky gut', the spaces between the cell walls are larger and they can allow larger molecules of bacteria, waste matter and undigested food through into the bloodstream. Your immune system views these substances as 'alien' and acts to eliminate them. Antibodies are made against these proteins derived from previously harmless foods, and these antibodies can trigger an inflammatory reaction next time the corresponding food is eaten.

If you have an actual food allergy, you will get an immediate and usually severe reaction, but intolerances may have less clear-cut symptoms, manifesting in different parts of the body over the longer term. They are generally not life-threatening but can make you feel unwell. The only way to diagnose an intolerance is to avoid food you suspect for a period of months and see if symptoms clear up.

Clogged-up colon

A common symptom of toxin overload and a diet that is dependent on processed foods is a clogged-up colon. Normally the colon produces just enough mucus to move faeces along, but when toxins, drugs or stress irritate your colon, it produces excess mucus which can bind with starchy waste materials to make hardened faeces. These become impacted in nooks and crannies in the colon, meaning that the villi cannot absorb nutrients so efficiently and the gap through which waste material has to pass becomes narrower. The build-up becomes a breeding ground for bacteria and parasites (such as tapeworms and flukes), and you

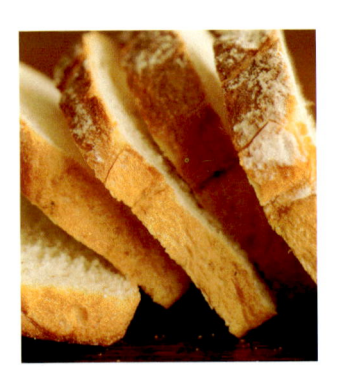

Many people in the West are wheat-intolerant and will get bloated after eating it.

become constipated. In some people, a hard mass can actually be felt in the lower abdomen. They will probably suffer from flatulence, as the trapped food ferments, giving off gases and sulphur-containing compounds which give that characteristic smell.

Another problem with a clogged-up colon is that the longer waste material sits around without being eliminated, the more chance there is that the toxins in it will be reabsorbed by the body. Some people have faecal material in their colons that has been there for several years!

Stools diagnosis

You can check your stools, according to the following list, to see how healthy your gut really is.

- Eat some sweetcorn to test how quickly food is moving through your gut. You should be able to spot undigested husks when they come out the other end. This should take 24 hours or less.
- Do your stools float? This is good, but if they are so buoyant that you have trouble flushing them away, your liver is out of balance.
- How do they smell? Very smelly stools are a sign that your colon is clogged up and waste products are stagnating in there.
- How many wipes does it take to clean your bottom? More than three wipes and you are producing too much mucus, which means your colon is irritated. (This is also the case if you leave skid marks on the loo.)
- If your stools are tiny, hard pellets, your liver is congested.
- Stools should be a walnut colour. If yours are very light-coloured, it means that you are having trouble digesting fatty foods.
- Thin, shreddy stools are another sign of a clogged-up colon.
- Loose stools could be caused by a bug, or they could be a sign that your spleen is exhausted.

1 How toxic are you?

Fatty liver

Toxic compounds, such as alcohol, solvents, heavy metals, paracetamol, penicillin and hormones, are processed by the liver in two stages. First of all, they are changed into an intermediate form which is even more toxic, before they can bind to an amino acid or nutrient that will help their elimination in bile. If the process is interrupted, because the liver has so many other substances to deal with, the intermediate toxic compounds can circulate in the blood causing all kinds of damage.

Alcohol is broken down by the liver to acetaldehyde – a similar chemical to formaldehyde which is used to embalm dead bodies.

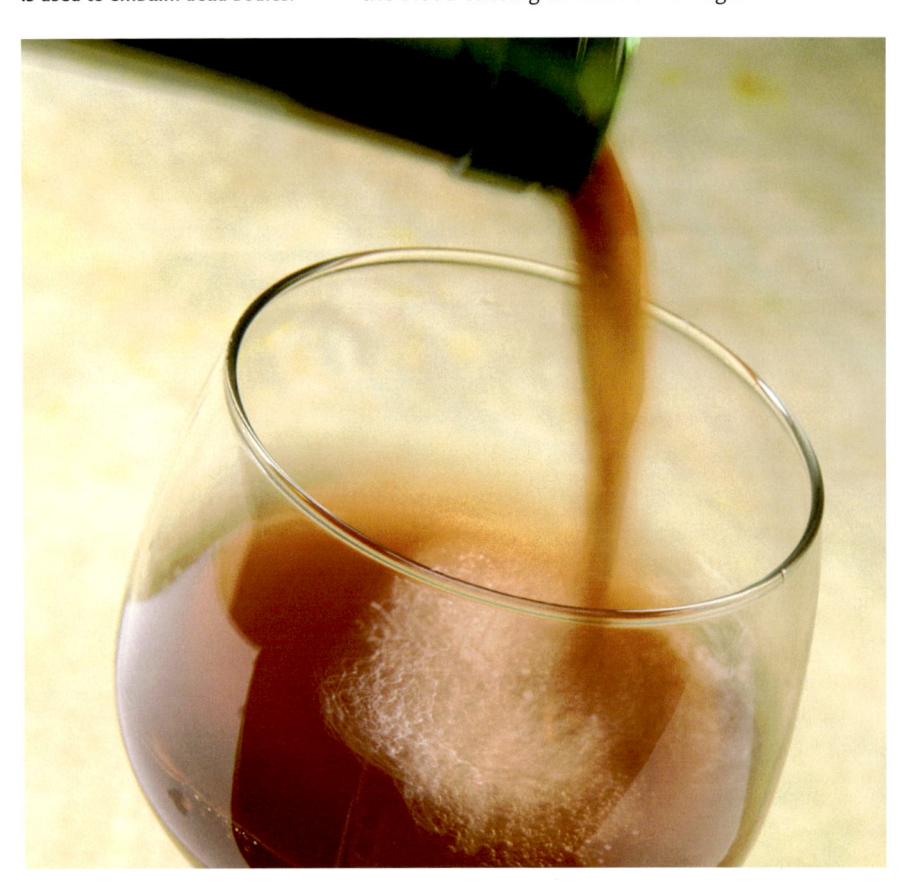

If the liver is not getting the substances it needs to make bile, you will have trouble digesting food, particularly fatty foods. Bile can become congested with filtered elements and will get backed up in the bile ducts. In this case, you will not be able to metabolize fats and will gain weight, and toxins and their by-products will remain in your circulation.

Alcohol is broken down by the liver to acetaldehyde, a toxic compound that leaches vitamins B and C and causes the kidneys to excrete more fluid, along with zinc, magnesium and potassium. The classic hangover symptoms are caused by dehydration, but this can be fixed by drinking lots of water to rehydrate. On a more sinister note, the free radicals formed by acetaldehyde will be attacking cells and causing them to degenerate (see page 40).

A liver that has to deal with excess toxins, particularly alcohol, will begin to form fatty deposits inside its cells. Fatty liver is now recognized as the most common cause of abnormal liver function tests in the West, with around 20 per cent of the UK population suffering from it. Long-term exposure to acetaldehyde causes scarring of the liver tissue leading to cirrhosis. There has been a sharp rise in liver cirrhosis deaths in the UK over the last 20 years, more than doubling for people in Scotland and increasing by two-thirds for men in England.

However, if you stop the damage before it reaches the cirrhosis stage, the liver can break up its fatty tissues and regenerate itself remarkably well. Even if you just give up drinking for a week or a month, you give your liver a chance to catch up on the backlog; every drinker, no matter how moderate, should do this from time to time.

must know

Drinking

More than one in five men and almost one in 10 women binge drink every week, consuming more than eight units of alcohol a day for men and more than six for women. A unit is 300ml (½ pint) beer, a 125ml (4fl oz) glass of wine or a measure of spirits. Excessive alcohol intake is the most common cause of sudden fits in young men. A woman's risk of getting breast cancer rises by six per cent for each extra drink she has on a daily basis, and she is at more risk of brain damage from alcohol than men.

1 How toxic are you?

Kidney stones

Stones form in the kidneys when urine stays too long in the system, so drinking plenty of liquid is essential to keep them eliminating waste efficiently. Urine should be a pale straw colour and you should produce at least 2 litres (3½ pints) per day, on around five to six trips to the lavatory. Any darker than this, and any less volume, and you are not drinking enough water, so toxins are sitting around longer than need be inside you.

Weight problems

If your digestive system and liver are not functioning effectively, you will find it difficult to keep your weight down. A toxic liver that cannot metabolize fat and cholesterol just dumps them back in the bloodstream. Many toxins are then stored in body fat, and the more fat you have, the more waste you will collect. Conversely, the more toxins in your system, the fatter you are likely to be.

According to the World Health Organization, 76 per cent of British men aged between 30 and 69 years are overweight, compared with 65 per cent 10 years ago; 69 per cent of women are overweight compared with 55 per cent in 1995. One in five men and women are categorized as clinically obese. As a nation, we are just getting fatter and fatter, making us much more at risk of life-threatening diseases, such as diabetes, heart disease and cancers.

Fat stores, particularly abdominal fat, become metabolically active like an organ in their own right, pumping out hormones that just exacerbate the situation. A waist measurement of more than 90cm (36in) in men – 80cm (32in) in women – is

> **must know**
>
> **It's in the eyes**
> Look at your eyes to see how well your liver is functioning. Are the whites white or a dull cream or yellowy colour? Do you have dark shadows under your eyes? Both are signs of a liver that is struggling to eliminate toxins.

Being overweight has mental as well as physical side effects; it is often associated with low self-esteem, depression and performing less well in exams.

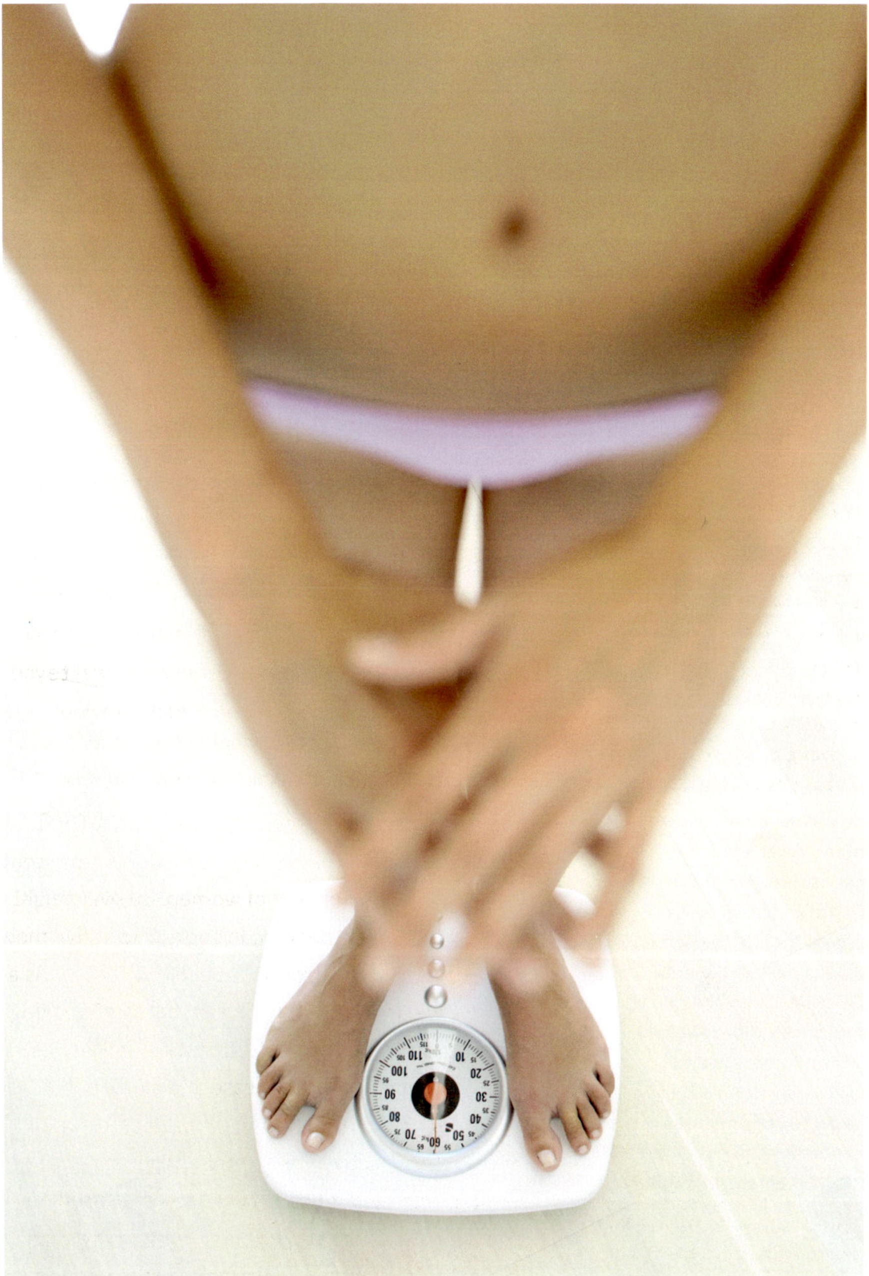

1 How toxic are you?

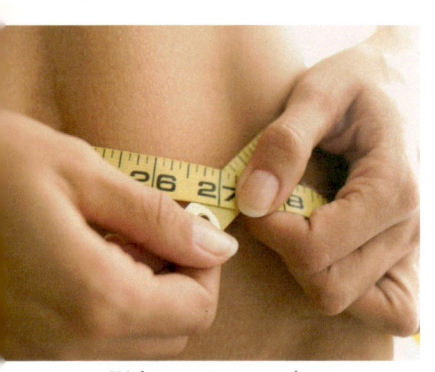

Waist measurement is an important indicator of your risk level for many illnesses.

associated with an increased risk of experiencing metabolic complications.

Waist-to-hip ratio
This is a recognized clinical method of evaluating abdominal fat. The waist is measured at the narrowest point, whereas the hips are measured at the widest point, and then the waist measurement divided by the hip measurement gives the waist-to-hip ratio. If it is higher than 1.0 for men and 0.85 for women, you have too much abdominal fat and are putting your health at risk.

Cellulite
This is the orange-peel dimply flesh that women tend to get on their hips and thighs. Men get it too, but it is usually not so obvious because they have more muscle tissue to disguise it. Cellulite is caused by sluggish circulation, which means that lymph fluid and toxins accumulate between connective tissues. Hormone supplements, such as the Pill or HRT, can contribute, as can stress, a sedentary lifestyle, lack of exercise and binge eating.

Skin problems
The skin is a mirror that shows not only how well your elimination organs are working, but also the level of toxins in your body and whether you are lacking vitamins and minerals in your diet. If your skin is very reactive, prone to spots, blotches, rashes, eczema or psoriasis, you probably need to clean out. Toxicity will also make you look more tired and wrinkly, and your skin tone will be yellowy or greyish rather than clear and glowing.

> **must know**
>
> **Cancer and excess weight**
> The American Cancer Society produced a study in 2003 which found that the more overweight a person is, the higher their chance of developing many types of cancer. Excess weight was a factor in 20 per cent of cancer deaths in women and 14 per cent in men. Obese women are two to four times more likely to get endometrial and kidney cancer, twice as likely to get pancreatic cancer and 46 per cent more likely to get colon cancer.

Compromised immunity

Canadian researcher Hans Selye found back in the 1940s that when a person is exposed to a new toxin they have not encountered before, they respond with physiological shock. Blood flow to the area is decreased while the body works out how to deal with the toxin and adapts to it. When the system is overloaded with new toxins, the adaptation process is less successful and a range of symptoms can set in. Selye noted an increase in allergies, psoriasis, arthritis and asthma, plus hormone fluctuations and mental problems ranging from depression to learning difficulties.

While your body is struggling with a range of day-to-day toxins, the immune system can become compromised, making you more prone to picking up opportunistic infections, such as colds, flu and herpes cold sores. If you feel you get more than your fair share of bugs, it might be worth thinking about taking steps to reduce your toxic load.

Do you need to detox?

There are many, many more effects of toxins on the body and not enough space to list them all here. If you are still unsure whether you have a toxic overload which is dragging down your general

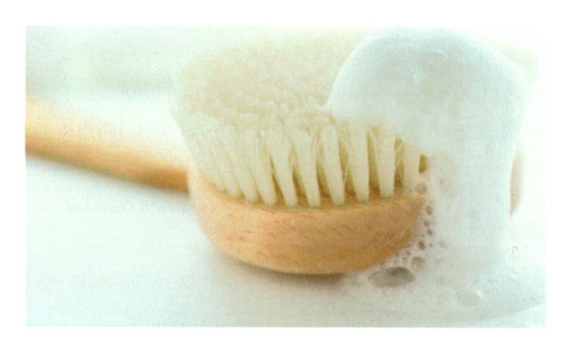

> **must know**
>
> **Infertility**
> According to a study in *The Lancet*, average sperm count in British men fell from 113 million per millilitre in 1940 to 66 million in 1990. Between eight and twelve per cent are now functionally sterile, with a sperm count of less than 20 million per millilitre. Women who have had repeated miscarriages typically have partners with low sperm counts. Studies have shown that poor nutrition plus excessive alcohol and caffeine intake are the main cause; oestrogens in the water, our food and the environment also play a part in this.

Regular body brushing can help break up cellulite deposits.

1 How toxic are you?

Tongue diagnosis

Practitioners of Traditional Chinese Medicine (TCM) will always check your tongue when making a diagnosis, because it is a good indicator of general health. A healthy tongue should be pale red with a thin white film, and smooth and moist. Is yours like this, or do you recognize the following?

- A thick yellow coating means your bowels aren't working efficiently.
- A thick white coating on the tongue means there is too much mucus in the system and not enough beneficial bacteria in the gut.
- A crack down the middle of the tongue means a weak stomach. If you have this, you are probably prone to bloating.
- Watch out for cracks, teeth marks and red patches on the tongue. Depending on location, they indicate that an organ is underfunctioning. The right side of the tongue shows the performance of the gall bladder, the left side is the liver, the middle is the stomach and spleen, while the back of the tongue mirrors the kidneys, intestine, bladder and womb.

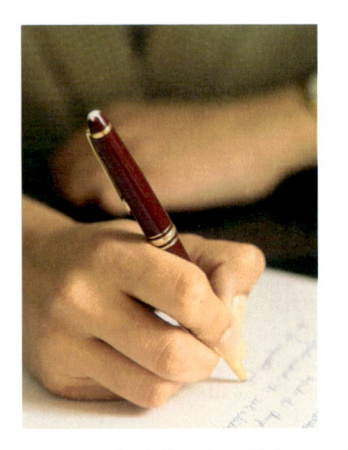

Keeping a food diary, in which you list what you have eaten and how you felt afterwards, can help you to self-diagnose any allergies and intolerances.

physical and mental functioning, answer the following questions and add up the number of yes's.

Examine yourself

- Have you taken more than two or three doses of antibiotics in your life?
- Do you often feel sleepy after eating a meal?
- Do you ever get cravings for specific foods?
- Are you gassy? Do you burp, fart or get bloated after eating fatty foods?
- Do you often get a bitter taste in your mouth?
- Do you have bad breath or smelly body odour? (Ask a close friend!)
- Do you suffer from joint stiffness or muscle weakness?
- Do you often feel fatigued for no reason?

- Do you frequently wake between 1am and 3am and are not sure why?
- Do you have trouble sleeping?
- Do you find it hard to concentrate?
- Are you worried about your memory?
- Do you think you get drunk more easily than your friends?
- Are you depressed for no obvious reason?
- Do you get more colds than your contemporaries?
- Do you often get a stuffy, blocked-up nose?

FOR WOMEN
- Have you been trying unsuccessfully to get pregnant?
- Do you suffer from PMS or pronounced menopausal symptoms, such as hot flushes?

FOR MEN
- Do you have problems getting and maintaining an erection?
- Has your partner had trouble conceiving a baby?

Self assessment

If you have answered 'yes' to even one of these questions, then the chances are that you have a toxic burden which is affecting your health. Basically, even people who live on remote islands cannot avoid pollutants altogether, although some are more reactive than others. There is controversy in the medical profession about the notion of 'detoxification', as some of the extreme methods can do more harm than good, but in the next chapter, we will take a look at how a gentle detox programme could help you start to shift some of your toxins and make you feel much, much better.

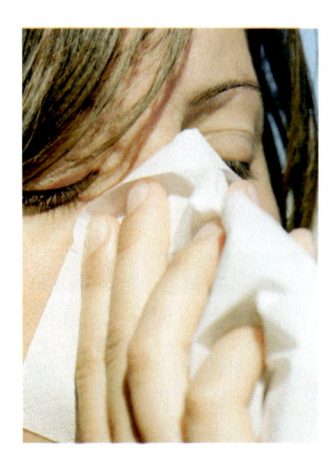

Sneezing and nasal congestion are often symptoms of allergies.

want to know more?

- For some shocking facts, read *Not in the Label* by Felicity Lawrence.
- Don't leap straight into a drastic detox diet. Follow the guidelines in Chapter 2 to prepare your system first.

weblinks

- For information on digestive disorders and pesticides, look at:
www.digestivedisorders.org.uk
www.gn.apc.org/pesticide trust
www.chem-tox.com/infertility

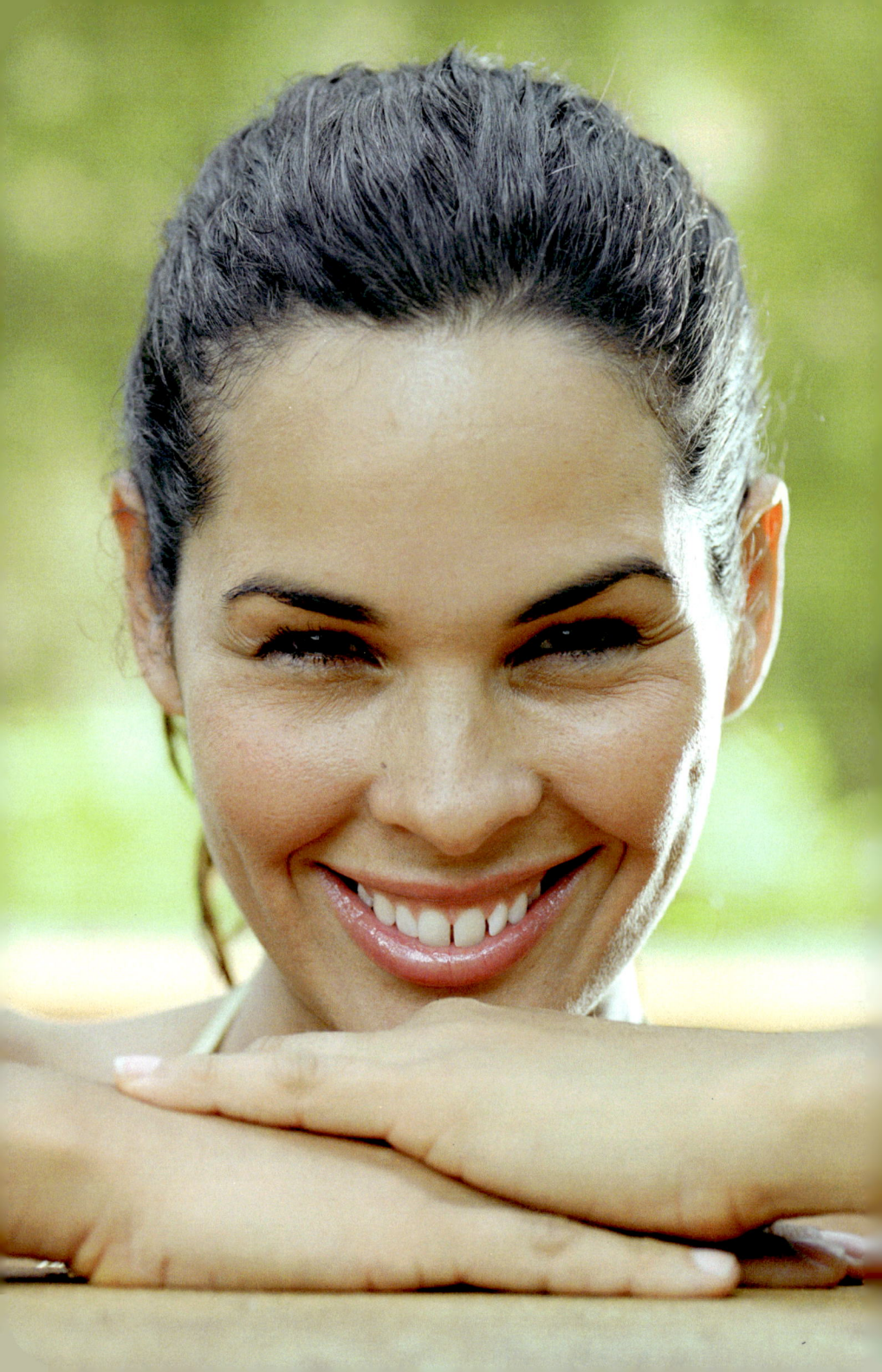

2 How detoxing works

Detoxing should never be entered into suddenly, without preparation or after a period of excess. Indeed, many medical experts advise against it altogether because of the harm it can do if your body is not ready to deal with the mass release of its stored toxins. However, follow the gentle, step-by-step approach in this chapter and you can begin to cleanse your system, but you must be aware that you will not get rid of 40 years' worth of ingested toxins with just seven days of good behaviour. Get ready for the long haul if you are serious about improving your health.

2 How detoxing works

Body shock

If you have never tried detoxing before, start at the beginning of this chapter and then work your way through slowly. Those of you who have detoxed before and don't have any serious bad habits can skip to the seven-day plan (see page 45).

must know

Thyroid cancer
The thyroid gland, in the front of the neck, is particularly susceptible to radioactive fallout; thyroid cancers increased by 8,000 per cent in children who lived within 100 miles of Chernobyl after the nuclear disaster there. They are also increasing generally, with the incidence more than doubling in the UK over the last 30 years. A 1955 report in the *New England Journal of Medicine* showed a 400 per cent increase in cancers of the thyroid in San Francisco during the period when their water was fluoridated.

Cut out bad habits

Some detox programmes would have you cutting down overnight to a diet of raw vegetable juices accompanied by their recommended vitamin and herbal supplements. They require you to go cold turkey on caffeine, alcohol, wheat, dairy, salt, sugar, processed foods and many other toxin-laden or difficult-to-digest substances.

It's plans like these that have given detoxification a bad name in certain medical circles, because they would make you feel very ill if you tried them. A lifetime's worth of pesticide residues, drugs and other poisons stored in the fat cells is suddenly broken down and released into the bloodstream, causing all kinds of unpleasant symptoms. These can seriously compromise your immune and nervous systems and interfere with the action of your thyroid gland, and you would have been much better off staying as you were.

A balanced diet

Another criticism that the medical establishment fires at detox diets is that they are lacking in protein and essential nutrients that the liver requires in order to metabolize food. In Chapter 3, we'll look at how to select your detox foods and drinks to keep your diet balanced. Quick-fix detox diets, like crash diets, are not successful methods of losing weight, because when your body is deprived of food it goes into starvation mode and will retain all the calories it can to supply energy. When you start eating normally again, your metabolism will still be programmed to retain calories and so you could put on weight very rapidly. The first step in this gentle detoxification programme is to cut out any bad habits, such as smoking, excessive drinking of alcohol or caffeine, use of street drugs or over-the-counter medications.

WARNING: Don't stop taking any prescription medication without discussing it with your doctor.

must know

Street drugs
Detox programmes for coming off heroin and other opiate-based addictions should be closely supervised in specialist clinics, where withdrawal symptoms can be alleviated (see page 189 for contacts).

Each type of fruit and vegetable has its own unique combination of healthy phytonutrients.

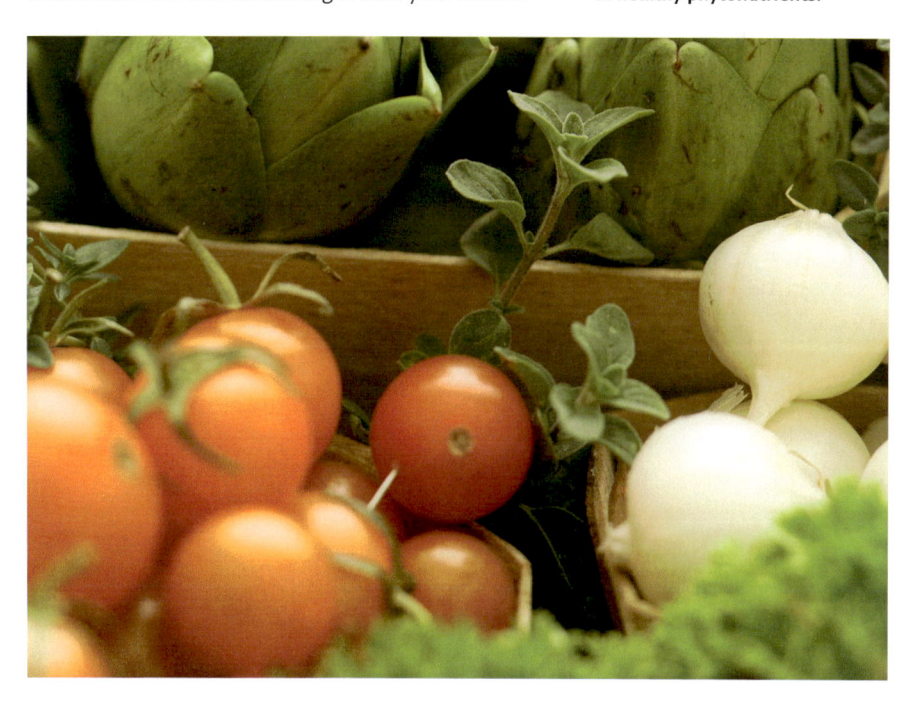

Body shock | 35

2 How detoxing works

must know

Sleep
Inadequate sleep lowers our immune response. Several studies have shown that missing even a few hours a night on a regular basis can decrease the number of 'natural killer cells', which are responsible for fighting off bacteria and viruses. This will come as no surprise to those who suffer from insomnia and find that they succumb to colds and other illnesses much more frequently than their partners who sleep through the night.

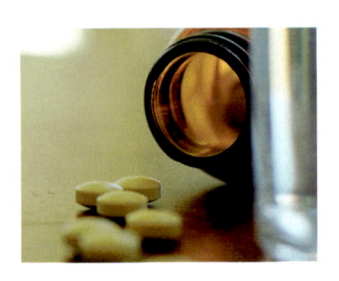

Above: If you take pills regularly, discuss with your doctor if they are really necessary.

Opposite: The National Sleep Foundation says that adults need seven to nine hours sleep a night to function at their best.

Smoking

If you are ready to quit the evil weed, there are dozens of organizations, books, tapes, herbal remedies and complementary therapies that can be of use. For more information, turn to the Need to Know More? section (see page 189). Oat straw, a concentrated source of B vitamins which is available from health food shops and alternative chemists, can help reduce cravings and quell the irritability that often accompany the first nicotine-free days.

Alcohol abuse

If you regularly consume more than two units of alcohol a day (for women) or three (for men), or if you ever drink more than six units in one session, you are putting your health at serious risk. One in three heavy drinkers will die in middle age because of drinking, even though they and their friends might not consider themselves to be 'alcoholics'.

Seeking help

Cut out alcohol completely at least seven days before you plan to detox. Your liver will start to recover straight away, from the first alcohol-free day. If you have trouble cutting out alcohol, you may need help. Talk to your GP or call Alcoholics Anonymous. A Chinese remedy called kudzu, which is available from alternative chemists or TCM centres, is useful for combating cravings when you give up alcohol. Take 150mg three times a day, and drink lots of water.

Over-the-counter drugs

An estimated 30,000 people in the UK are addicted to OTC medications, with painkillers at the top

Body shock | 37

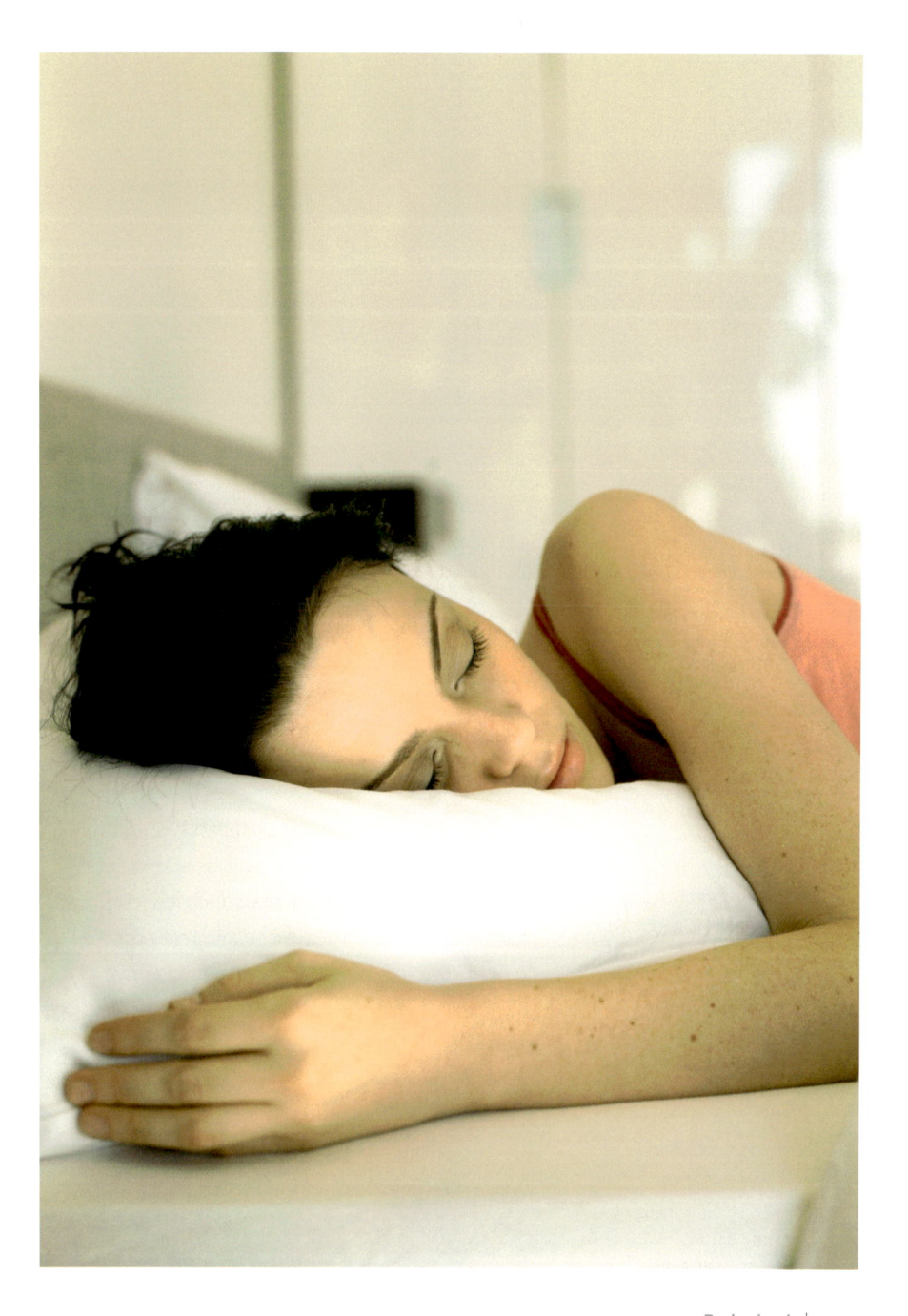

2 How detoxing works

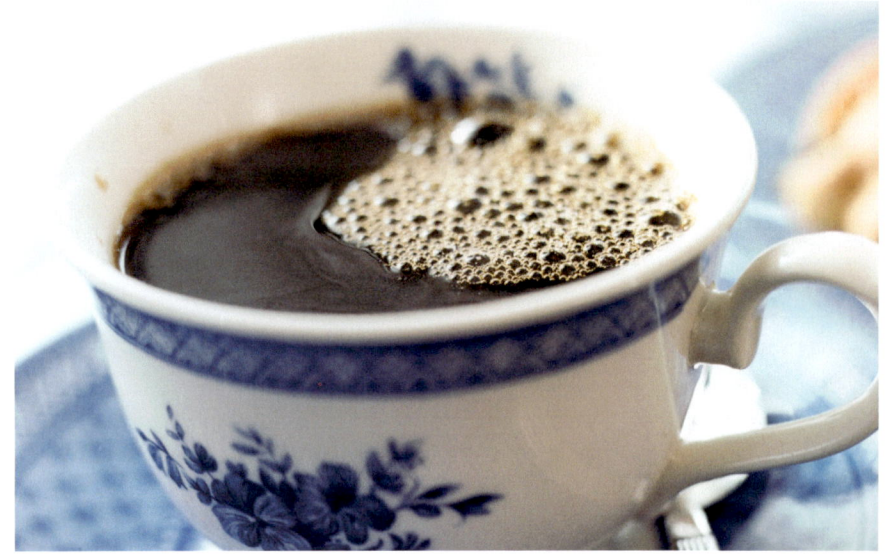

Coffee ages the skin and can weaken your immune system.

> **must know**
>
> **Sugar highs**
> Are you a sugar addict? Sweets cause blood sugar peaks and troughs which give you mood swings and energy dips as well as affecting the performance of your liver, pancreas and spleen. Substitute sugar with natural sweeteners like honey or fructose, and cut right back on the quantities.

of the list and cough medicines second. There are many side effects of this kind of dependency. One study, for instance, found that the regular use of ibuprofen doubles your risk of suffering a heart attack and substantially increases your risk of stroke. The long-term misuse of painkillers can lead to physical and psychological dependency, chronic constipation, headaches, nausea, liver dysfunction, all kinds of gastrointestinal disorders, depression, mood swings, chronic lethargy and restless limbs, to name but a few.

The warnings on packets state that patients taking these drugs for longer than three days should see their doctor, so do heed this and get treatment for any underlying illnesses that are causing your symptoms. Talk to a herbalist, homeopath or naturopath if you would like to investigate a holistic path to feeling well enough so that you no longer need OTC drugs (see page 189 to find a therapist).

Caffeine withdrawal

Caffeine is right up there with nicotine as one of the most addictive substances around, and, just like nicotine, it can produce severe withdrawal symptoms when you cut it out. Remember that caffeine is found in fizzy drinks, chocolate and painkillers as well as in tea and coffee.

If you are used to having three or more doses of caffeine a day, you will probably experience withdrawal symptoms when you give it up which could include headaches, irritability, an inability to concentrate, cravings, anxiety, fatigue, a runny nose and, possibly, nausea. Don't rush to the medicine cabinet for some paracetamol, though, or you'll undo the good work you've started. Use rosemary, peppermint or lavender aromatherapy oils applied to the temples, the pulse points behind earlobes and the back of the neck to relieve headache and nausea. Chamomile tea is also good for the relief of mild to moderate headaches, and Bach flower essence Rescue Remedy can help (see page 130).

If you are having a real problem with caffeine withdrawal symptoms, you may need to take this stage more slowly. Switch from coffee to green or black tea, which still has caffeine but also contains bioflavonoids and catechin, a substance that protects against heart disease and cancer and boosts the metabolism. When you are accustomed to drinking tea instead of coffee, cut back gradually by replacing a cup a day with herbal teas – there are lots of delicious varieties you can try. Don't attempt to start a detox programme until you have sorted out your caffeine dependence or you will give your system too much to cope with.

> **must know**
>
> **Caffeine content**
> Caffeine makes the heart pump blood faster and has a diuretic effect. It can reduce fatigue and increase your concentration, but you quickly build up tolerance and need ever-greater doses to achieve the same effect. Strong coffee has around 200mg per cup, while strong tea has just 80mg, cola has 45-75mg and cocoa has just 10-15mg. Regular caffeine addicts can get withdrawal symptoms after just a few hours without their 'fix'.

2 How detoxing works

Antioxidants v. free radicals

must know

Grapefruit
Citrus fruits are all great sources of vitamin C, but you should avoid grapefruit when you are detoxing. It contains a substance that slows down the body's ability to process the toxins in alcohol, air pollution or prescription drugs. When you are next scanning the menu in a cocktail bar, watch out for drinks containing grapefruit juice and alcohol and give them a wide berth.

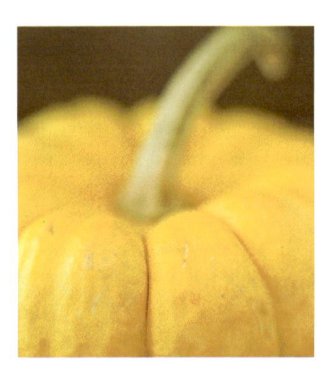

Free radicals are unstable molecules which are created in the body as a result of some normal metabolic reactions. However, more are generated by smoking, drinking alcohol, environmental pollutants, taking antibiotics or paracetamol, or burning body fat while on a weight-loss diet. Free radicals have a negative electric charge and they try to neutralize this by colliding with other molecules so they can pass on their spare electron in a process known as oxidation. Excess oxidation damages cell material and causes a number of degenerative problems and diseases, including atherosclerosis (furring and hardening of the arteries), heart disease, premature ageing and cancer.

The main defences against free radicals in the body are substances called antioxidants that can neutralize their negative electric charge before the damage is done. Antioxidants are nutrients taken in through the diet, and as you prepare for a detox it is crucial that you increase your antioxidant intake. By boosting your intake of foods containing the four major antioxidants at the same time as you are cutting out alcohol and caffeine, your detox preparation will be well under way.

Carotenoids
These are found in yellow, orange, red and dark green fruits and vegetables, including carrots, tomatoes, spinach, sweetcorn, mangoes, peaches, watermelons and pumpkin. By reducing the oxidation of fats circulating in the blood, they diminish the risk of heart disease, cancers and cell damage, especially to the eyes.

Pumpkins are full of alpha- and betacarotene, vitamins C and E.

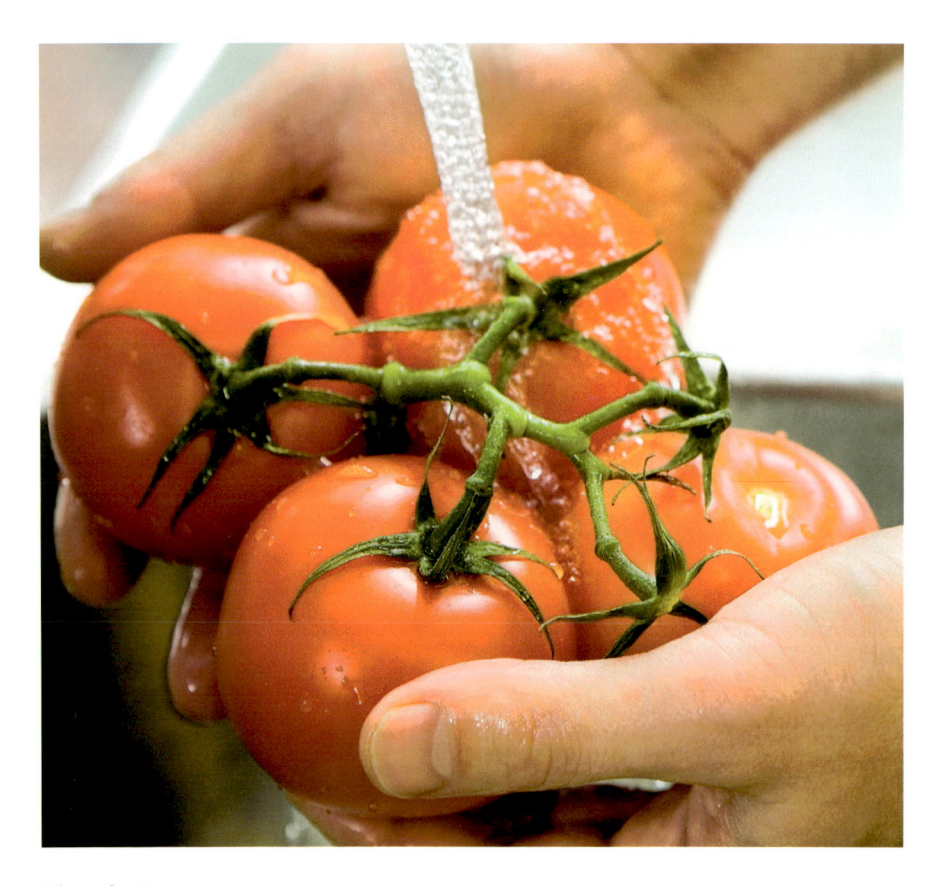

Vitamin C

As well as being a powerful antioxidant, this vitamin prevents the conversion of nitrites (found in many processed meats and other pre-packaged foods) into carcinogenic nitrosamines. Vitamin C boosts the immune system, protecting against a wide range of bacterial and viral diseases, cancers and heart disease. It also helps to maintain sperm quality and prevent skin ageing.

Rich sources of vitamin C include blueberries, kiwi fruits, blackberries, rosehips, oranges, red peppers, papaya, cantaloupe melon, broccoli and tomatoes.

As well as vitamin C, tomatoes contain lycopene which helps to protect us against several different types of cancer.

2 How detoxing works

Vitamin E
Food sources include avocado, eggs, nuts, seeds, whole grains, oily fish and broccoli, and should always be eaten raw where possible, because cooking destroys part of the vitamin E content. This crucial vitamin is the most important anti-ageing nutrient and it does seem to counteract some of the negative effects of pollution and heavy metals, while boosting the immune system and reducing the risk of heart disease and cancer.

Selenium
This valuable mineral binds to harmful toxins like mercury, arsenic and cadmium and strengthens the immune system's ability to destroy cancerous cells. You'll find it in Brazil nuts, fish, poultry, whole grains, mushrooms, onions, garlic, broccoli and cabbage.

Avocados contain 14 different minerals that the body needs, including iron, which helps in the formation of red blood cells.

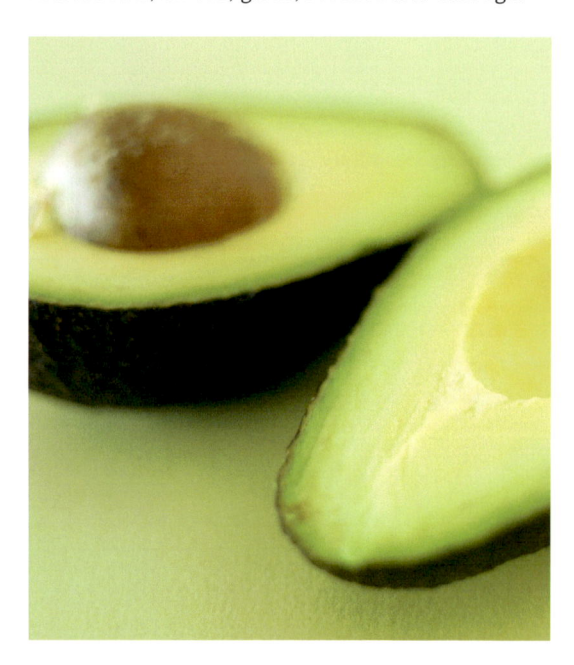

Bump up your fibre

Did you pass the stools test on page 23? You should have bowel movements at least once a day and pass well-formed, walnut-coloured, non-sticky stools that float on the surface of the water but flush away easily. In the UK, studies show that most people get only about 12g of fibre a day, although the minimum recommended level is 18g and many experts say that 35g is optimum. Almost all of us would benefit from including more fibre in our diets, and when you're preparing for a detox it's essential to ensure your bowels are moving food through efficiently, so you can get rid of all the toxins that are excreted from your cells

Fibre in common foods

1 bowl whole oat porridge (not instant)	8.5g
Half a cup of kidney beans	7.9g
Half a cup of chickpeas	7g
1 bowl of muesli	4.3g
1 medium apple	3.8g
1 handful of dried prunes	3.4g
1 medium pear	3.3g
1 large handful of sunflower seeds	3g
1 medium corn on the cob	2.5g
1 medium raw carrot	2.5g
1 slice of high-bran bread	2.4g
1 large handful of Brazil nuts	2g
1 portion of broccoli, boiled	1.4g
1 fist-sized portion of brown rice	0.6g

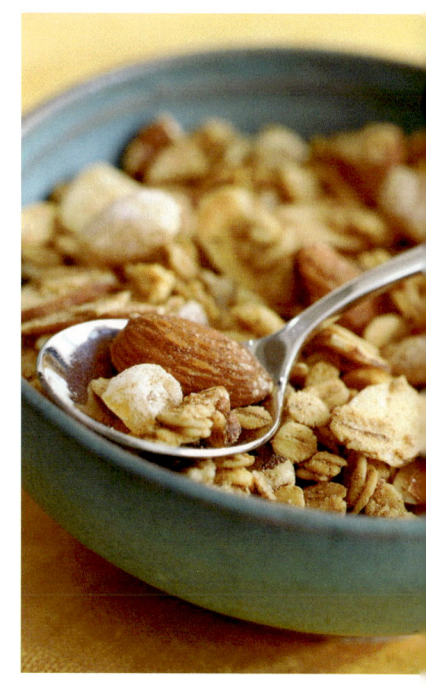

Try making your own muesli, adding millet flakes for extra fibre. And, as they are gluten-free, they will not irritate the walls of your intestine.

2 How detoxing works

> **must know**
>
> **Irritable bowel syndrome**
> This condition causes intermittent abdominal pain, wind, nausea, bloating and alternating bouts of constipation and diahorrea. It is interesting to note that in 80 per cent of cases, IBS sufferers are found to have an overgrowth of fungi, bacteria or parasites in their guts. Detoxing can help, under the supervision of a qualified therapist, and because there appears to be a link with stress and anxiety, relaxation techniques can be beneficial.

instead of re-absorbing them. At least a week before a detox, start eating new sources of fibre until you can pass the stools test.

Add fibre gradually. If you add too much too quickly, you could experience bloating, wind and abdominal discomfort. Increase the amount of water you drink to eight 225ml (8fl oz) tumblers a day (see page 66 for advice on which water) to wash down and bulk up the fibre in your diet.

Choose a week

Choose one when you don't have important work commitments, as you may find your concentration is not up to par, and avoid weeks with a lot of social engagements as it will be hard to resist the pressure to join in. You may get more tired than usual, so you will need plenty of early nights. Don't choose a week when you have a major sporting commitment, such as a tennis tournament. Your performance will be affected and you could make yourself ill.

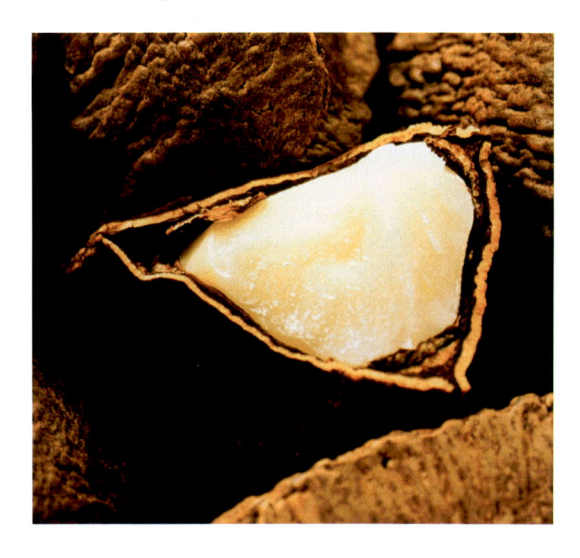

Just one large Brazil nut contains the recommended daily intake of selenium.

7-day detox

If you have managed to give up alcohol and caffeine and bump up your antioxidant and fibre intake without experiencing more than mild side effects, then you are ready to try a proper detox, and a 7-day plan is a good starting point.

Before you start

Here are some general guidelines before you start your 7-day detox, which will help you to plan ahead and have a greater chance of success.
- Buy a wide range of the foods listed on the detox shopping list (see page 69)
- Decide which herbs and supplements you want to take (see pages 116–121) and buy them either by mail order or from a good complementary chemist.
- Buy a skin brush, Epsom salts and any oils, flower essences, foot patches or other treatments you are planning to use at home (see pages 126–131).
- Book appointments for any complementary therapies that you would like to aid your detox methods (see Chapter 6).

Rules of the 7-day detox

- No caffeine or alcohol are allowed. Substitute herb teas, dandelion root coffee and fresh juices.
- No dairy foods are permitted on the 7-day detox. Milk and cheese increase mucus production and are difficult to digest. Lactose is a common food intolerance. You can replace milk with almond milk, rice milk, oat milk or soya milk. Sheep's and goat's products are easier to digest if you really cannot do without dairy.

must know

Who can detox?
- Ask your doctor if you have any ongoing health condition for which you are receiving treatment, e.g. diabetes, heart disease, hypoglycaemia, liver or kidney problems, thyroid problems, cancer or stomach ulcers. Do not detox if one of the following applies to you:
- If you are about to have, or just had, surgery.
- If you are on warfarin, blood pressure drugs, antidepressants or birth-control pills.
- If you are pregnant or breast-feeding.
- If you are under 18.
- If you have a mental illness, e.g. depression, anxiety, bipolar disorder, schizophrenia, eating disorder.

2 How detoxing works

> **must know**
>
> **Seasons to detox**
> In traditional Chinese Medicine, spring and summer are the best seasons for a detox. Winter is a time to rest and recuperate, eating a wholesome and warming diet. Spring is the best time to deep-cleanse the liver and gall bladder. Light, cleansing foods should be eaten in summer, and in the autumn the focus is on the intestine, lungs and skin, as you eat harvest vegetables, such as pumpkin and squash.

- No wheat or gluten-containing grains, such as rye, which have an acid effect on the digestion. This means no bread, pasta or white rice. Choose oats, brown rice, millet and quinoa instead.
- No meat or poultry, because of the antibiotics and food additives they contain. For protein, choose plant sources, organic eggs, tofu or oily fish from organic (non-farmed) sources.
- No processed or ready-made foods whatsoever. Everything should be fresh and cooked without salt, sugar or sweeteners. Use fresh herbs for seasoning.
- Eat three meals and two snacks every day, making sure that you have something to eat every three hours. Most of your food will be vegetables and fruit, whole grains and plant proteins. There are sample menu choices for a 7-day detox on page 76.
- Do make sure that you get at least 20 minutes of exercise every day.
- Drink 2 litres (3½ pints) of water a day and have cups of herbal (non-caffeine-containing) teas whenever you feel like them.
- Dry-brush your skin before a shower or bath at least once a day and, if you can bear it, follow your bathing routine with a cold shower (see page 149).

What can you expect?

Headaches and fatigue are normal in the first few days of a detox. Some people even feel as though they are coming down with flu, a syndrome that complementary therapists call a 'healing crisis'. What is happening is that old chemicals stored in fat tissues are being released into the bloodstream: antibiotics, pesticides, food additives, heavy metals and other waste products. Some people break out in spots as their body sheds toxins through the skin; others get constipation, diarrhoea or bad breath with the change in digestive routine; yet more feel giddy and nauseous. Take it easy and keep drinking 2 litres (3½ pints) of water throughout the day. If the symptoms don't pass in four days, consult a doctor to rule out any underlying illness.

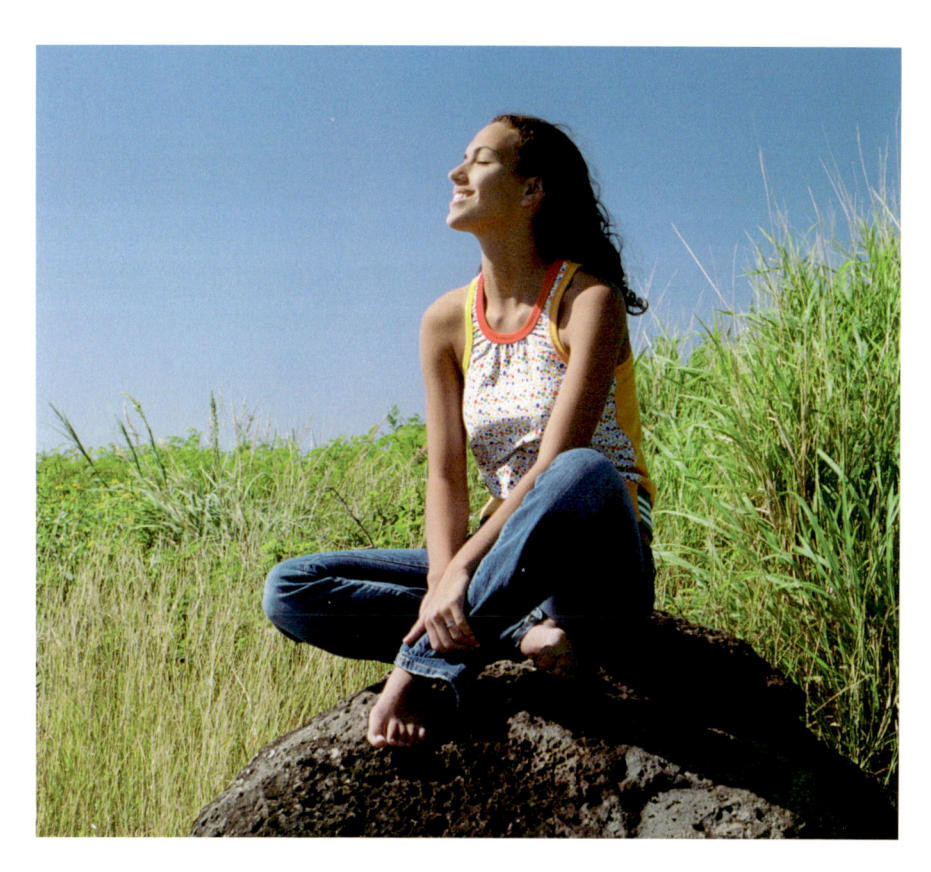

Although you won't purge a lifetime's worth of toxins during your first-ever detox, you will have made a significant difference. Next time you try a detox, the healing crisis won't be so severe and will probably not last so long. A 7-day detox is a step

Choose a period to detox when you don't have any stressful commitments in your life.

2 How detoxing works

towards better health but you should find that by the end of it, your skin looks clearer and glowing, and you feel more energetic and clear-headed. Your bowels and liver should function more efficiently and you'll have given your immune system a mini-boost.

Weight loss

Most people lose weight when they detox, because they are avoiding fats, sugars and all the other foods and drinks that pile on the calories. If you return to your previous eating patterns after seven days, you will soon replace any kilos you have lost. If you have more weight to lose, continue eating according to detox rules, but reintroduce organic meats and poultry, wheat and dairy, as described below. Stay off processed and packaged foods and keep eating fresh as much as possible. You probably will not need to calorie-count or reduce your portions – few people overeat on such a healthy diet. The only danger is slipping back to old ways of eating.

Coming off your 7-day detox

Don't wolf down a four-cheese pizza and a bottle of Pinot Grigio on day 8 or you will feel unwell. Keep eating the same kinds of food as on the detox but gradually introduce organic poultry, then red meat, goat's or sheep's cheese and wholegrain bread.

If you suspect you are intolerant to a particular food or foods, test yourself by leaving five days between reintroducing each new food and watching for a reaction. If you experience bloating, headaches, skin rashes, joint pain or unusual symptoms, you may decide to exclude the culprit from your diet for a longer period. All traces of a food will be removed

---

must know

Hot lemon
Some people swear by the benefits of kick-starting their system first thing in the morning with a drink of freshly squeezed lemon juice (from unwaxed organic lemons) added to hot water. Just sip it slowly and feel it cleansing your gut ready to face the day. You may find this precipitates the day's first bowel movement. Leave half an hour after this drink before eating your detox breakfast.

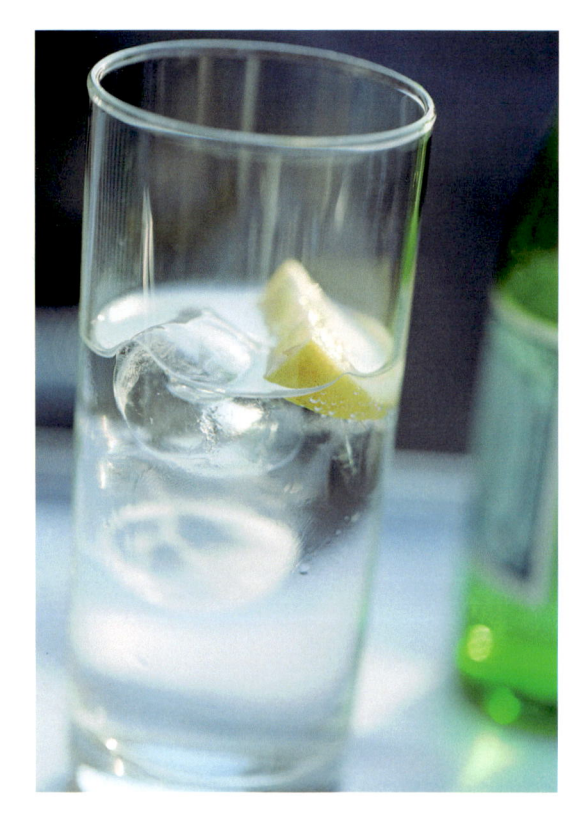

Limonene, which is found in lemons, helps the immune system to destroy cancer cells.

from the body within two months, so reintroduce it after three months to see if you now tolerate it. Sometimes intolerances pass, especially if you have been helping your system by unburdening some of the toxic load and stimulating healthy organ function.

Hang onto as many good habits from the detox as you can fit comfortably into your lifestyle. Opt for liver-supporting foods. If you miss coffee, reintroduce a single cup of organic coffee in the morning, but check for any symptoms of dependence developing, e.g. jitteriness and inability to concentrate without it. Most detox experts advise that you repeat your detox every six months.

2 How detoxing works

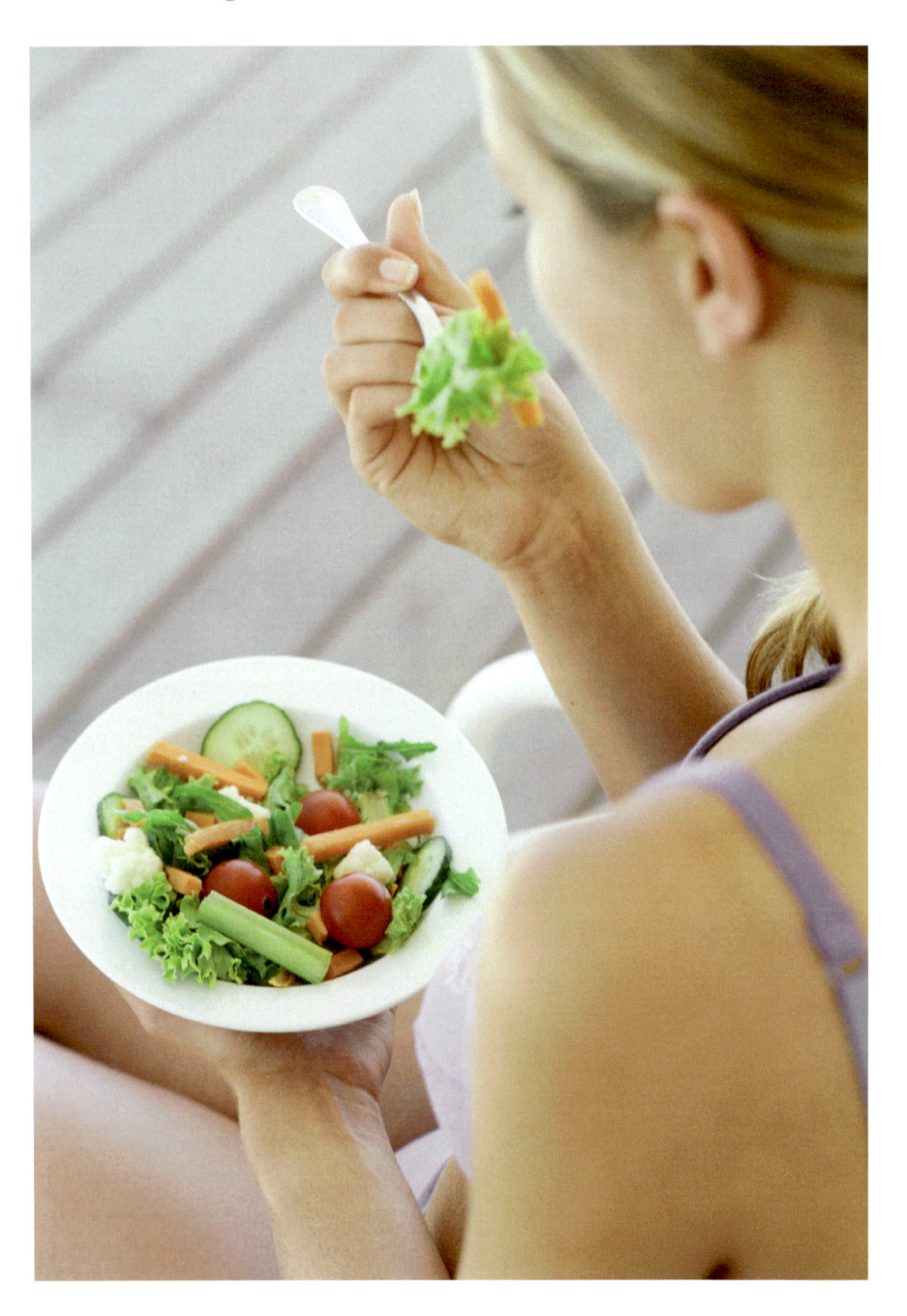

30-day detox

Different experts advocate different lengths of time for detox programmes. Seven days is a good starting point and if this worked for you, why not try a longer detox to shift more of the toxins? Some plans are geared to 14 days, others to 28 or 30, but they will follow similar rules to the ones already described.

Diet plan

When you undertake a longer detox, say 30 days, you either have to follow an exact menu plan worked out by a nutritionist or educate yourself very carefully about nutrition so as to avoid deficiencies. For example, when you are not eating meat, poultry or dairy, you need to work harder to make sure you are getting the amino acids your body needs to grow and repair tissue. Eight of these must come from our food, and they are known as 'essential' amino acids. A 'complete protein' contains all eight. Meat, poultry, fish, eggs, dairy products and tofu are complete proteins, as are quinoa and amaranth. Grains, pulses, beans, nuts, seeds and green vegetables are incomplete proteins but if they are eaten in the correct combinations, they can make up a complete protein. Mixing brown rice with beans is a good tip.

Making up complete proteins

Here are vegetarian dietary sources for the eight:

- L-lysine: potatoes, soya products, lima beans, yeast.
- Methionine: garlic, onions, lentils, beans.
- Phenylalanine: almonds, avocados, bananas, lima

must know

Lactose intolerance
This results from a deficiency in lactase, the enzyme responsible for digesting lactose in milk. It is more common in those with certain ethnic backgrounds. It affects more than 50 per cent of people of Native American, Afro-Caribbean or Indian origins, but only three per cent of Caucasians. Young children may get temporary bouts of lactose intolerance after they've been treated with antibiotics or had a dose of gastroenteritis.

Opposite: You should include as many different colours in salads as you can, to get a wide range of nutrients in your diet.

2 How detoxing works

beans, pumpkin seeds, sesame seeds.
- Tryptophan: barley, brown rice, soya beans, peanuts.
- Leucine: wheatgerm, oats.
- Isoleucine: wheatgerm, nuts, seeds.
- Threonine: nuts, beans, seeds.
- Valine: found in most plant foods.

Benefits

The advantages of a 30-day programme are that your body has time to adapt and become used to a more healthy way of operating. You will cleanse more of the toxic load and should look and feel much better when you finish. It is recommended that you follow a structured detox plan to ensure you get all the nutrients you need to stay healthy. Once again, the real benefit of the detox will come if you manage to retain lots of the good habits you've learned and stick with a fresh-food diet long term.

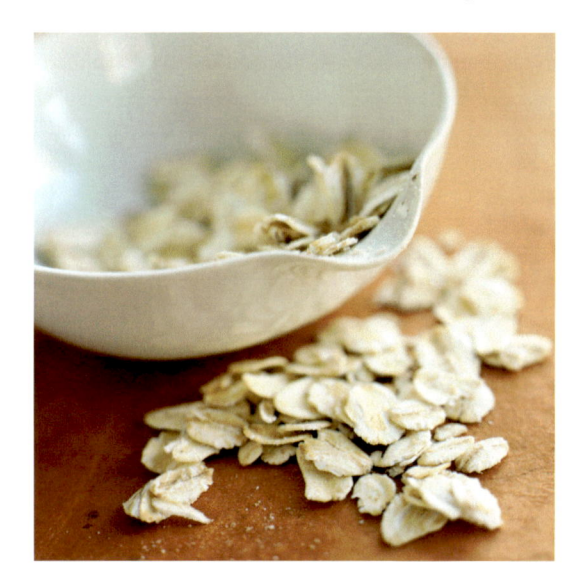

must know

Food combining
Some nutritionists believe that it is easier for our digestive systems to break down foods if we don't eat a protein and a carbohydrate at the same meal. It is worth trying if you suffer from digestive problems. Eat protein and salad or vegetables for one meal a day, then eat grains, pasta or cereals with vegetables for another, and only eat fruit on its own at least 30 minutes after a meal.

Oats are rich in B vitamins and fibre, both of which can help the body to cope with stress.

One-day or weekend detox

One- to three-day detoxes generally involve fasting – cutting out food altogether and surviving on water alone, or water plus freshly prepared fruit and vegetable juices. Some juice fasts allow you to have raw vegetables as well.

Fasting

Needless to say, you won't find many GPs or mainstream medical specialists who approve of this drastic kind of measure, and you certainly should not undertake a fast unless you are in an extremely good state of health to start with. Don't choose fasting as your first-ever type of detox. Wait until you have tried a few 7-, 14- or 28-30-day ones and are no longer experiencing side effects from them. Build up gradually to a fast, as the body can go into panic mode if you suddenly make a huge change in your eating habits. If your system thinks you are starving, it will retain all the fat (and toxins) it can, rather than releasing fat cells for elimination.

The rules of fasting

- Start preparing for your fast several weeks in advance, cutting out caffeine, alcohol, wheat, meat and dairy. Get used to eating mainly plant foods.
- Don't ever fast if you have any kind of chronic illness or have recently recovered from a viral or bacterial infection.
- The first time you fast, only do it for a day. Stay at home if possible because you may feel very faint and weak. You certainly shouldn't drive or operate heavy machinery.

must know

History of fasting
Many cultures have advocated periodic fasting to give the digestive system a rest and cleanse the body. In the Western medical tradition, Hippocrates, Galen and Paracelsus were all fans of periodic fasting. Ayurvedic practitioners and yoga teachers in India recommend it for its physical and mental benefits. Native Americans go to sweat lodges while fasting and Scandinavians developed saunas as their method of sweating toxins from the body during a fast.

2 How detoxing works

- Drink 2–3 litres (3½–5 pints) of water on your fast day, and a selection of juices made from organic fruits and vegetables. Fruits are good for cleansing, while vegetables help to repair the cells.
- Don't do a water fast for longer than a day except under the supervision of a qualified practitioner, and don't do a juice fast for longer than three days. You are not getting the nutrients you need to stay healthy and your detox will soon become counterproductive, because the liver needs protein in order to carry out its detoxification processes.
- Wean yourself gradually back onto solids after the fast has finished, starting with soups, oat porridge and easy-to-digest dishes (any of the recipes in Chapter 5 would be good).

Pomegranate juice is the new super-juice, with more antioxidants per glass than any other fruit juice.

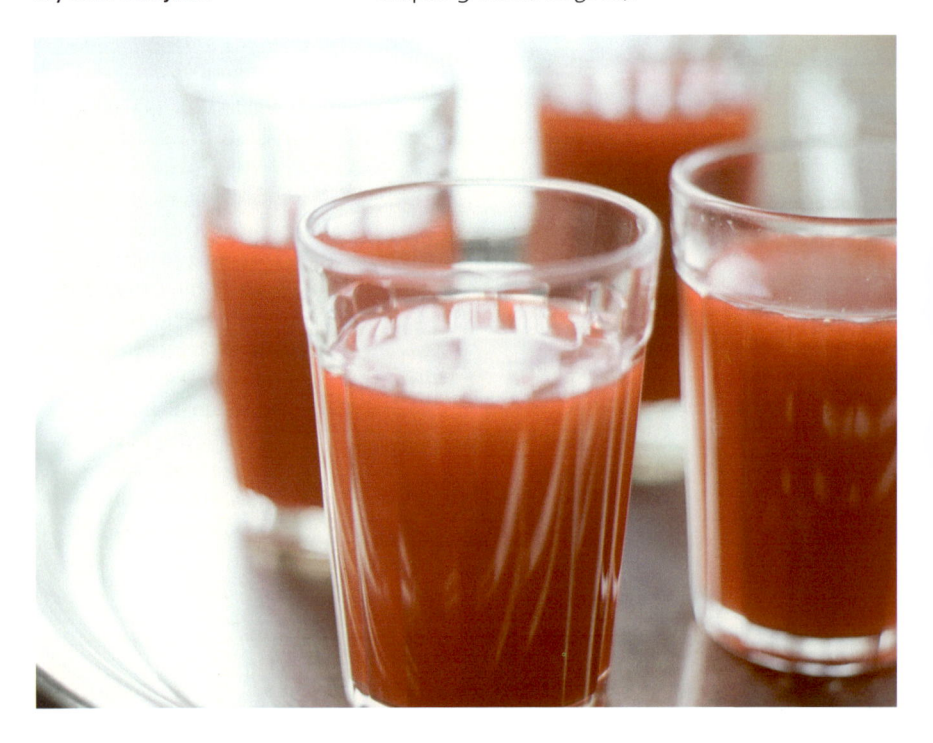

Long-term maintenance

Even the medical specialists who disapprove of detoxing agree that it is a valuable process if it helps to teach you healthy habits that you retain after the detox is over.

A healthy lifestyle

By retaining the healthy habits you acquired during your detox, you will experience ongoing health benefits. For instance, you will get fewer headaches and your skin will look better if you keep drinking 2 litres (3½ pints) of water a day. Your immune system should function more effectively if you stick with a diet full of antioxidant-rich fruits and vegetables, and you will have a better chance of avoiding heart disease and several types of cancer.

You should try to keep your fibre intake up at around 35g a day for healthy bowel function and to protect you against the increasingly common colon cancer. Keep skin brushing to hold the cellulite at bay and you will improve your circulation all round. Also, by cutting out the junk foods in your diet, you will have a much better chance of keeping your weight within a healthy band.

Mini-detoxes

Detox enthusiasts advise that you repeat it twice a year, but between times you can give yourself a boost by undertaking mini-detoxes where you give up alcohol or caffeine for a week but without necessarily following all the other rules. No doctor in the world could possibly object to that!

want to know more?

- See Further Reading on page 190 for books that can help you give up smoking and alcohol, plus a recommended detox diets list.
- There is a range of healthy detox recipes in Chapter 5.

weblinks

- For help on giving up smoking, log on to Narcotics Anonymous: www.ukna.org
- Alternatively, try the Action on Smoking and Health website: www.ash.org.uk
- Call Alcoholics Anonymous to find your nearest meeting: 020 7730 0009 www.alcoholics-anonymous.org.uk

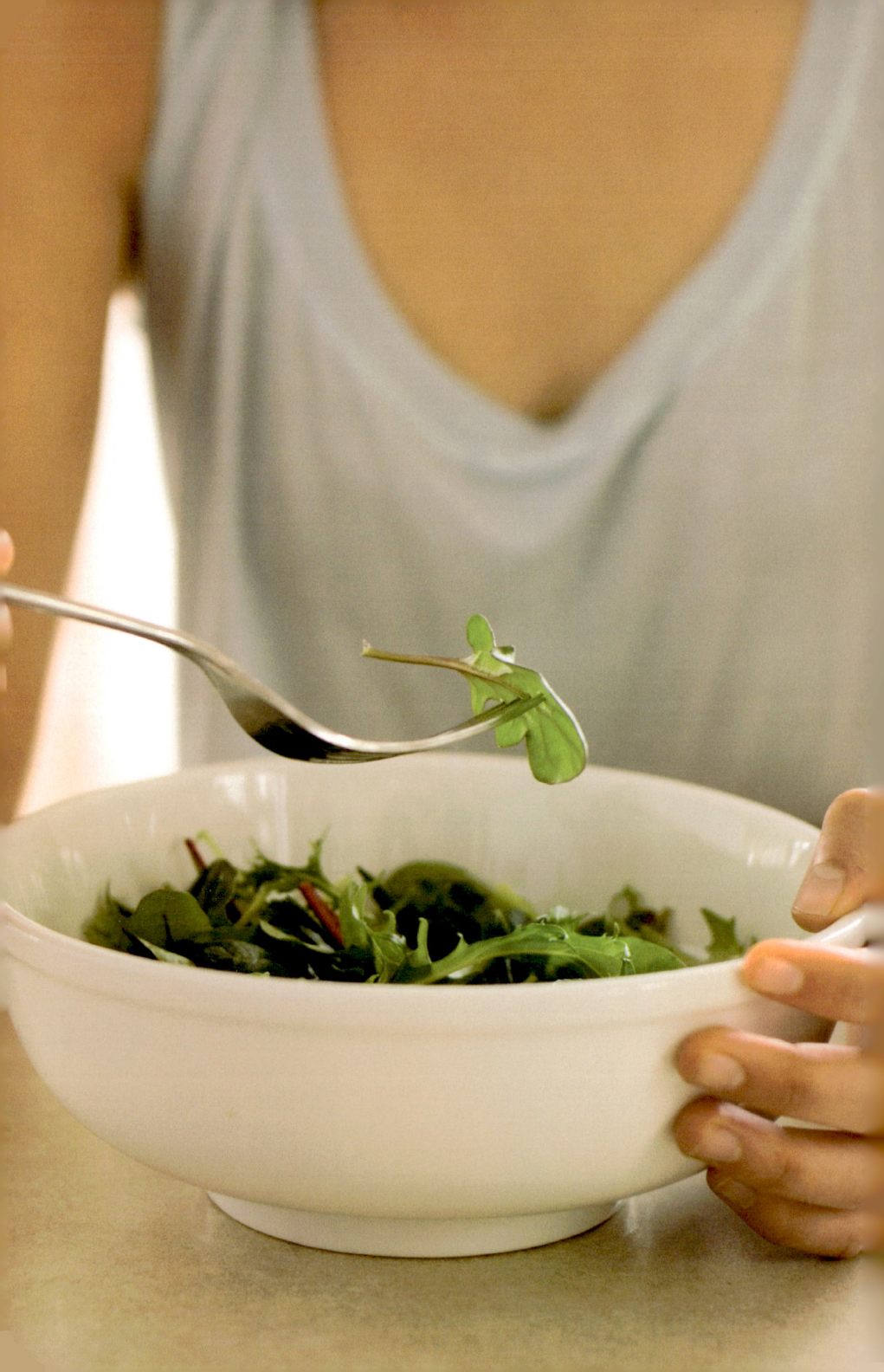

3 What to eat and drink

Detoxing isn't just about avoiding the foods and drinks that tax the liver and burden the digestive system; it's also about opting for fresh, natural foods that positively boost your metabolism and provide loads of health-promoting nutrients that strengthen your natural detoxification processes. The main aim of the diet is not weight loss, so do not start counting calories or jumping on the scales every day. The benefits will be measured in how well you look and feel at the end of your detox programme.

3 What to eat and drink

Clean up your diet

You should never go hungry when you are detoxing. Eat as much as you like. Have between-meal snacks. The only rule is that you stick to detox foods and drinks. If you have stocked your kitchen in advance, it should not be too hard.

must know

Money tight?
If you cannot afford to buy all organic, at the very least avoid the fruits and vegetables with the biggest toxin load when they are grown conventionally: strawberries, apples, cherries, apricots, blackberries, pears, raspberries, peaches, imported grapes, spinach, peppers, celery and potatoes.

Go organic

What is the point of going to a lot of trouble to cleanse the toxins from your system if you are simultaneously reintroducing new ones with every morsel you eat? By choosing organically grown foods, you can avoid the most harmful pesticides. The ones that are used on organic crops are strictly regulated and natural farming methods are used to control pests, such as crop rotation and the planting of anti-pest plants alongside crops.

Harmful chemicals
Some fruit and vegetable crops are treated with more harmful chemicals than others:

• Non-organic strawberries are covered in captan, a fungicide that has been linked to cancer, damage to the immune, nervous and reproductive systems, and birth defects.
• Non-organic apples contain diphenylamine, which some experts believe causes brain and nervous system damage, and thiabendazole, which may damage the reproductive system.
• Non-organic celery contains permethrin, chlorothalonil and acephate, all linked to cancer.
• Non-organic spinach will often have up to 40 harmful pesticides on its leaves.

Preparing fruit and vegetables
No amount of washing or peeling will shift these chemicals because the soil they were grown in, which has nurtured them, is replete with toxins. You should still wash and peel them but do not kid yourself that you are solving the problem.

Is organic more nutritious?
Researchers at John Hopkins University looked at the results of 41 studies over a 50-year period and concluded that on average organic food contained 30 per cent more vitamin C, over 20 per cent more iron, 30 per cent more magnesium and 14 per cent more phosphorus than conventionally grown food, as well as 15 per cent fewer harmful nitrates.

Although you will not eat meat on your detox, it is worth knowing that organically reared animals cannot be fed the growth enhancers and parasiticides that non-organic animals receive. Antibiotics are not given preventively and, if the animal gets ill and requires antibiotic treatment, it is removed from the organic herd. Their feed must be 100 per cent organic, with no genetically modified ingredients and no animal by-products. Finally, when the meat is sold, it should contain no artificial ingredients, food colourings or chemical preservatives.

Without going into gruesome details, pork is probably the most toxic of non-organic meats because pigs don't sweat out toxins in the way that some other animals can; and non-organic chicken can be seriously bad for your health with more than 60 per cent of factory-farmed birds infected with campylobacter from their own faeces, and more than 30 per cent infected with salmonella.

> **must know**
>
> **Brown rice**
> As well as being a great source of B vitamins, brown rice is good on a detox as a kind of 'pipe cleaner'. It travels through the gut, absorbing waste and then flushing it out at the other end. Try to choose short-grain rice for the best cleansing properties.

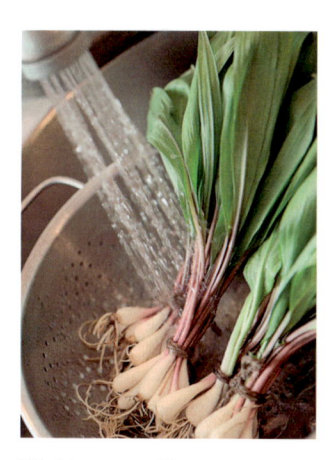

Washing vegetables removes the external layer of pesticides.

3 What to eat and drink

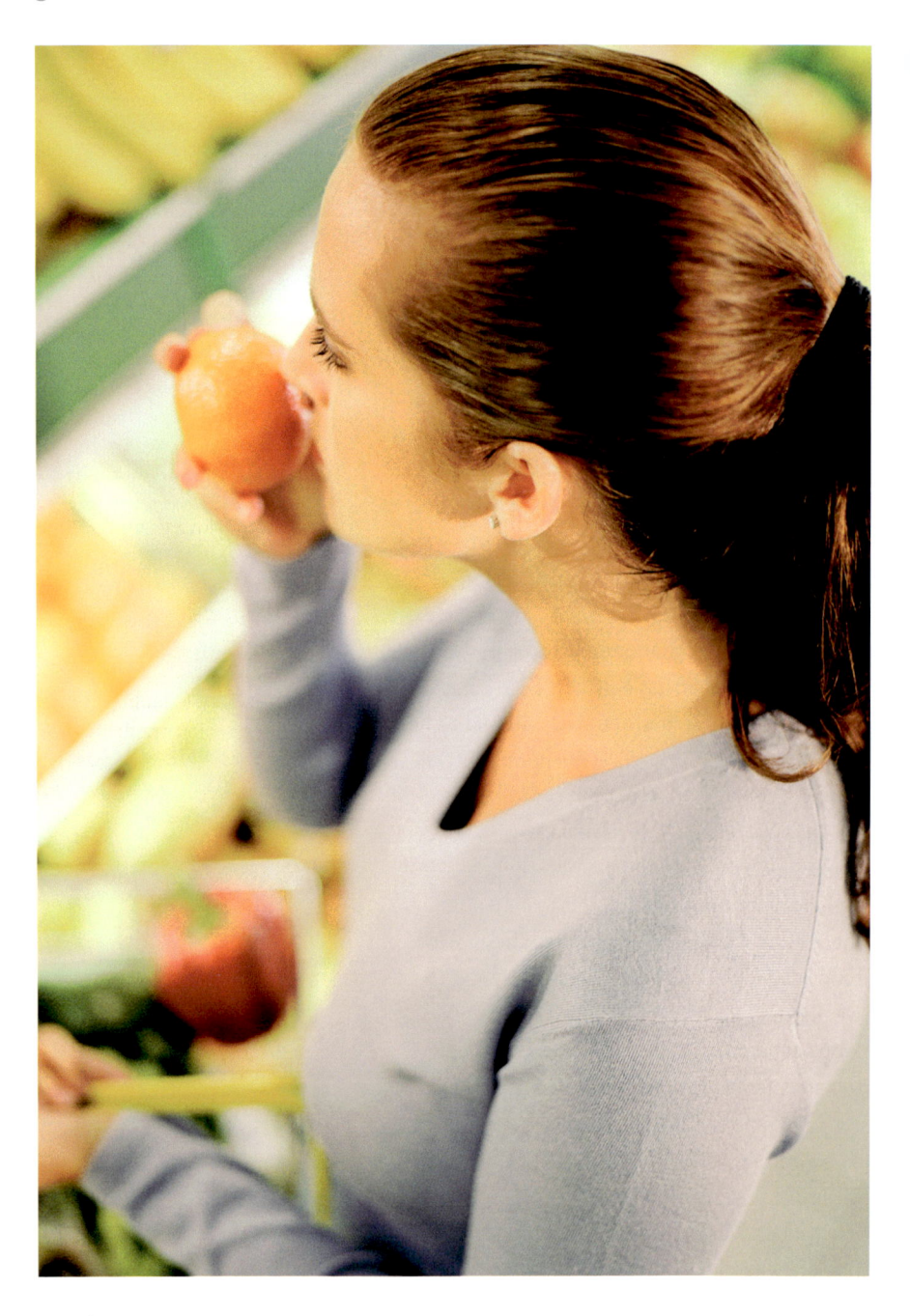

Help your liver to detox

Foods from the brassica family (cabbage, cauliflower, kale, pak choi, broccoli and Brussels sprouts) contain phytonutrients that are essential to the liver's detoxification processes and help the liver convert fat-soluble toxins into water-soluble substances which can be passed from the body in urine.

Liver healers

Sulphur-rich foods, such as garlic, onions, eggs and red peppers, help the liver to eliminate toxins in a process called sulphation. In Asian restaurants, you may be served a long, white radish called a Daikon after eating particularly fatty foods, because its high sulphur content helps the body to metabolize and digest fats. Certain other foods, some of which are listed below, are powerful liver healers because they contain key ingredients, and these should all be part of your detox programme. There are also a number of herbal supplements that boost liver function and will aid an effective detox (see page 119).

Artichoke hearts

These aid the secretion of bile, and they contain antioxidants known as flavonoids which protect the liver cells. Artichokes are a useful food for those people who have alcohol-related liver problems, and are a fantastic detox aid.

Asparagus

This is a good source of vitamin A and potassium, which the liver needs to detox, as well as being rich in folate, vitamin E and fibre.

> **must know**
>
> **Beating the booze**
> If you know you drink too much, it's best to stay away from other drinkers when you give up to help you resist temptation. Follow the advice on healing your liver, drink dandelion root tea and coffee, and take milk thistle (see page 119) and a good multivitamin supplement. Contact AA if you have trouble giving up.

Opposite: Smell fruits before you buy; the strongest-smelling will be the ripest ones.

3 What to eat and drink

Don't buy the artificially coloured pickled beetroot in jars; roast your own in the oven with a little olive oil and some thyme.

must know

Boost your kidneys
To help your kidneys flush away toxins, the most important thing is to keep up your water intake. Don't drink the 2 litres (3½ pints) all at once – spread them out through the day. Cranberry juice is a good kidney tonic, but look for one free of artificial sweeteners, or buy fresh cranberries in season. People who are prone to urinary tract infections should take regular cranberry supplements for their anti-bacterial properties, and should consider taking the herb buchu during a detox (see page 120).

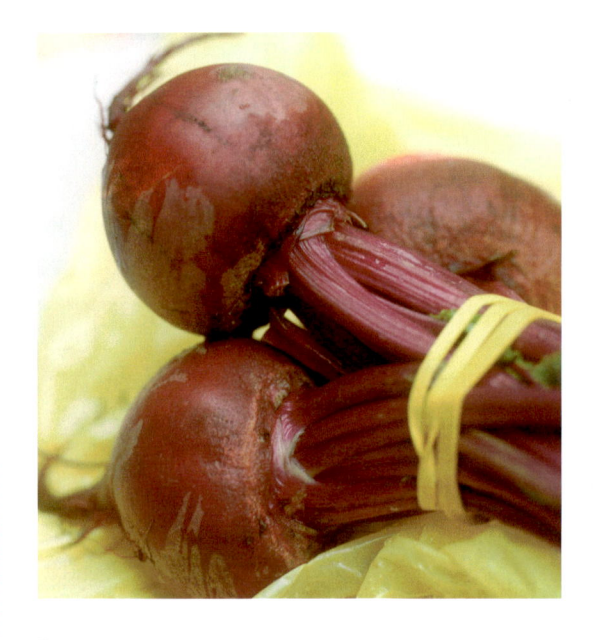

Beetroot
This contains betaine, which protects the liver from alcohol, and it also thins the bile and helps it to flow along the bile ducts more easily.

Dandelion roots
Dandelion roots contain inulin, which nourishes beneficial gut bacteria, stimulates liver function, and helps to lower blood sugar. You can buy dandelion tea and coffee in health food shops.

B vitamins
Contained in whole grains and pulses, such as oats, millet, chickpeas and brown rice, the B vitamins are essential in a liver detox. Vitamin B1 helps to deal with the effects of alcohol, smoking and heavy metals. B2 is used to produce glutathione. Vitamin B3 is needed for the breakdown of several toxins,

while B4 detoxifies the acetaldehyde byproduct of alcohol breakdown.

Magnesium

This essential mineral is found in dark green, leafy foods and is one of the key nutrients that your liver needs to manufacture enzymes for toxin breakdown. Choose bitter green leaves, such as watercress, rocket, chard, dandelion greens or mustard greens, to help your digestive enzymes and to provide the chlorophyll which purifies the blood.

Oranges, lemons and limes

These stimulate the production of glutathione and help the process by which the body eliminates sulpha drugs. Start finding some new ways to use

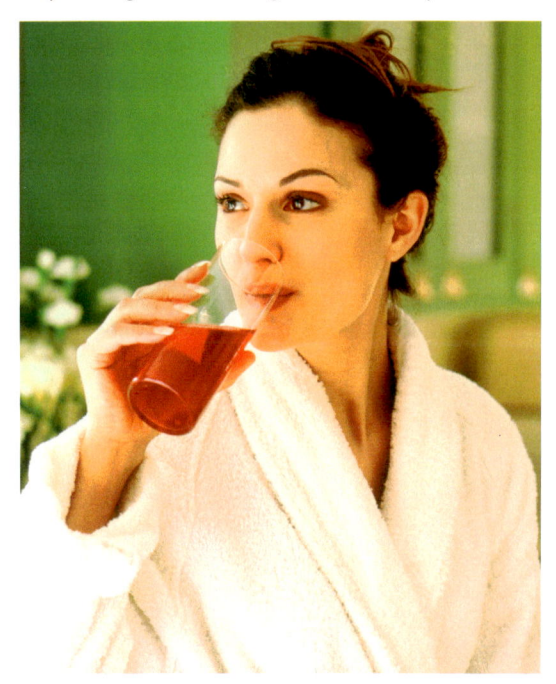

must know

Seeds
Pumpkin, sunflower, sesame, flax and alfalfa seeds are a concentrated source of vitamins, minerals and essential fatty acids. You can toast pumpkin and sunflower seeds in the oven to bring out the flavour, or soak the seeds in water before eating to make them easier to digest. Sprinkle them on soups, salads, stir-fries or casseroles, or on your breakfast cereal.

Make a fresh juice for breakfast, so you start the day with a burst of valuable vitamins.

3 What to eat and drink

must know

Seaweed
Vegetables that come from the sea contain more minerals than any other single food source, with 10 times as much calcium as milk, and eight times as much iron as you'll find in beef. Choose arame, nori, wakame, kelp, kombu, dulse and hijiki. Follow the cooking instructions on the pack or just throw strips into the pot when you're cooking beans, rice or casseroles.

Choose non-fat or low-fat yoghurt rather than whole-milk if weight loss is one of your goals.

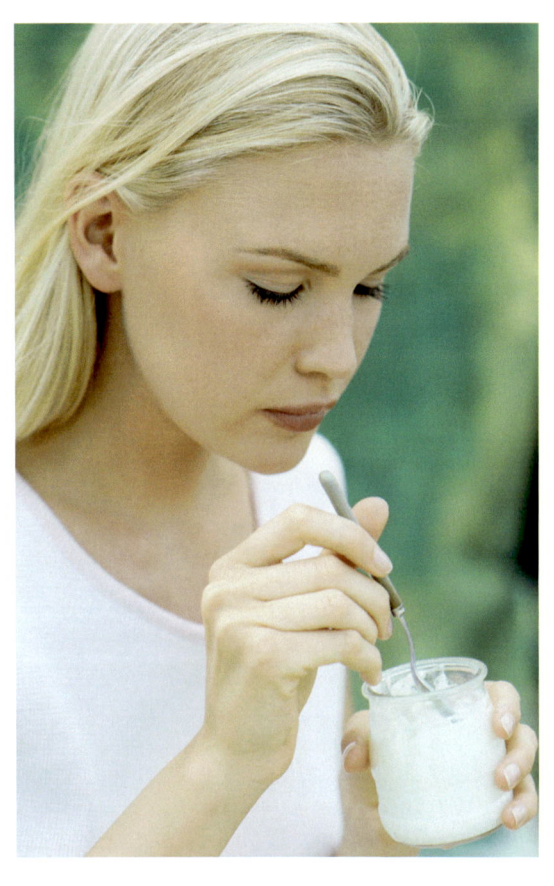

them; for example, adding some lemon juice to a cup of hot water to start the day; or mixing it with olive oil as a salad dressing; or squeezing some fresh orange and lime juice over a variety of crisp, wok-fried vegetables.

Turmeric
The key spice found in curries, giving them their distinctive yellow colour as well as flavour, turmeric slows down the first stage of detoxification in the liver but speeds up the second, so that you are

less prone to damage from the intermediate toxic chemicals and their associated free radicals.

Live yoghurt

Live yoghurt is a superfood that contains probiotics: beneficial bacteria that displace harmful toxins in your intestine. However, you must be sure that you get the right kind which has a high lactobacilli content. It should always say 'made with live and active cultures' on the label. If it has been frozen, or has artificial colours and fruit flavours added, you are on the wrong track.

Probiotic bacteria

These are fragile, and those that are found in 'bio' yoghurt which has been standing around on a supermarket shelf or in your fridge for a week or more will contain fewer live bacteria than freshly made cultures. If in doubt, you can buy probiotic supplements in health food shops – select one that supplies at least 1–2 billion colony-forming units (CFU) of acidophilus per dose.

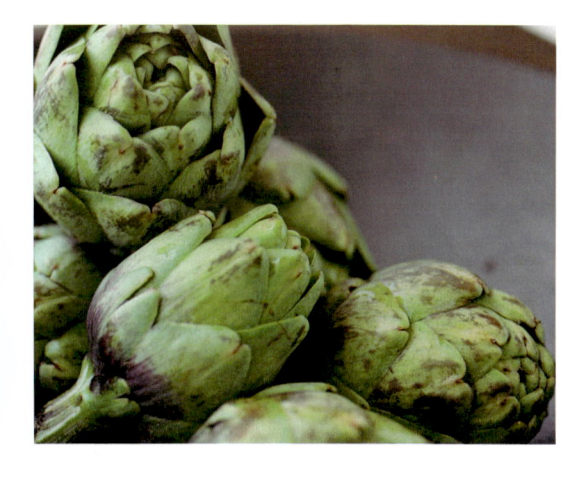

Some studies have found that artichokes can lower blood cholesterol levels if they are consumed regularly.

3 What to eat and drink

What kind of water?

Our blood is 83 per cent water, and it needs its supply of water to keep being replenished if it is to get rid of the toxins and waste products that your cells are shedding during a detox. But what kind of water should you drink?

> **must know**
>
> **Buying water filters**
> Look in your local directory for water treatment equipment suppliers, or ask your plumber to install a filter on your cold tap. For more water filter information and sales advice, see page 189.

Is tap water good for you?

Concerns about tap water include the risk of lead poisoning if your house was built before the 1970s and has lead piping. Even if it has been replumbed, the stop valve could be made of lead. Low levels of lead in the system have been linked to miscarriages, brain damage in children and poisoning in adults. If you think there might be lead in your water, contact the Drinking Water Inspectorate (see page 189).

According to some studies, adding fluoride to water suppresses thyroid function and causes the organs to stockpile aluminium, but several areas still add it to the water supply to protect against tooth decay. To find out what's in your local supply, you can ask for a water quality report from your local supplier.

Filtration systems

You can buy different kinds of filtration system to remove contaminants from your tap water.

Jug filters

These remove lime scale, chlorine and other impurities, but not hormones, fluoride or nitrates. The greatest improvement is taste, not quality. The filters should be changed monthly to be effective.

Plumbed-in sink filters
These claim to remove heavy metals, chlorine and 80 per cent of bacteria and pesticides. Once you have got past the installation cost, these are cheaper to run and more efficient than jug filters.

Reverse osmosis filters
The King of Filters is the reverse osmosis filter, filtering out between 95 and 98 per cent of minerals, chemicals, metals and bacteria, leaving you with a product that is purer than many bottled waters.

Bottled mineral water
This is convenient when you are out and about during the day. Always check that it is well before its sell-by date to avoid the risk of antimony poisoning from polyethylene terephthalate (PET) bottles and you should be fine.

> **must know**
>
> **Frequent urination**
> When you first increase your water intake to the recommended 2 litres (3½ pints) a day, or 8 x 125ml (4fl oz) glasses, you will find yourself trotting to the loo more frequently than usual, but within a week your system will get used to the extra liquid intake.

Reverse osmosis filters
It is scarey to think how many toxins are present in our water. Here is an example of what one reverse osmosis filter removes:

Bacteria 95%+	Ammonium 85-90%	Mercury 94-97%
Endrin 95%+	Bicarbonate 91-95%	Nickel 94-97%
Glucose 95%+	Bromide 88-92%	Nitrate 50-90%
Lindane 95%+	Cadmium 93-96%	Phosphate 97%
Methoxychlor 95%+	Calcium 93-96%	Potassium 88-82%
Phenol 95%+	Chloride 88-92%	Silicate 88-93%
Protein 95%+	Chlorine 95%+	Silver 88-92%
Pyrogens 95%+	Chromate 85-90%	Sodium 88-92%
Sucrose 95%+	Copper 94-97%	Strontium 93-96%
THM's 95%+	Cyanide 85-90%	Sulphate 93-96%
Toxaphene 95%+	Hardness 93-96%	Zinc 94-97%
Urea 95%+	Iron 94-97%	Fluoride 95%
Virus 95%+	Lead 95%+	
Aluminium 97%	Magnesium 93-96%	

3 What to eat and drink

Detox shopping list

If there are chocolate biscuits in the cupboard or some chilled Chardonnay in the fridge, the chances are you'll succumb during a weak moment and break your detox. Clear out 'banned' foods, give them away to friends or family, and replace with delicious detox foods to give you the best chance of success.

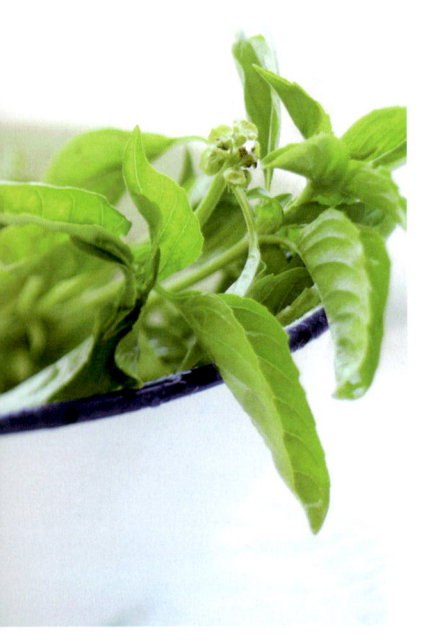

Explore the more unusual types of fresh herbs available at your greengrocer or in the supermarket and find out how best to use them.

Foods to avoid

It is so easy when you are pushing your trolley up and down the aisles of the supermarket to be tempted by all sorts of unhealthy and junk foods and to pop them in. However, you must learn to harden your resolve and opt for the healthy foods listed in the shopping list opposite while avoiding the foods featured below.

- Wheat products: including bread, wheat-based breakfast cereals, pasta, flour, noodles (except rice noodles), couscous, cakes, biscuits and pizza.
- Processed foods: including ready meals, ready-made sauces, condiments, stock cubes (unless organic), potato crisps, desserts, spreads, and anything that contains artificial additives. Always check the labels if you are unsure.
- Dairy products: such as milk, cow's cheese, cream, butter and normal, non-live yoghurts.
- All meat, poultry, game and non-organic fish.
- Caffeine: including black or green tea, coffee, chocolate, colas and other fizzy drinks, as well as painkillers.
- Sugars: including sweets, squashes, cordials and any juices except freshly squeezed.
- Alcohol.

Your detox shopping list

Fruits
Apples
Apricots
Avocado
Blackberries
Blackcurrants
Blueberries
Cherries
Greengages
Kiwi
Lemons
Limes
Lychees
Mango
Melon
Oranges
Papaya
Peaches
Pears
Pineapple
Plums
Pomegranate
Raspberries
Strawberries

Vegetables
Artichokes (canned and fresh)
Asparagus
Aubergine
Beetroot
Broccoli
Butternut squash
Cabbage
Carrots
Cauliflower
Celery
Courgettes
Cucumber
Green beans
Leeks
Mange-tout
Onions
Peas
Peppers
Pumpkins
Rocket
Salad greens
Spinach
Spring greens
Squash
Sweet potatoes
Sweetcorn
Swiss chard
Tomatoes (canned and fresh)
Watercress
All kind of fresh herbs: basil, mint, parsley, coriander, etc.

Grains
Amaranth
Brown rice
Buckwheat
Millet
Pasta made from corn, quinoa, rice or millet
Quinoa
Rice noodles
Rye flakes
Soba (buckwheat) noodles
Whole oat flakes
Wheatgrass, barley grass, alfalfa grass
Wild rice

Pulses (dried or canned)
Adzuki beans
Black-eye beans
Broad beans
Butter beans
Cannelini beans
Chickpeas
Flageolet beans
Haricot beans
Lentils, red or green
Red kidney beans
Sprouted beans

Nuts and seeds
Almonds
Brazil nuts
Cashews
Chestnuts
Coconuts
Dried fruit (unsulphured)
Flaxseeds
Hazelnuts
Pine nuts
Pumpkin seeds
Sesame seeds
Sunflower seeds

Breads and crispbreads
Wheat-free, yeast-free bread
Oatcakes
Rice cakes
Rye crackers

Spreads and dips
Guacamole
Honey
Hummus
Nut butters made without hydrogenated fats
Tahini

Protein
Organic free-range eggs
Goat's or sheep's cheese, including feta cheese and mozzarella
Organic oily fish (salmon, mackerel, herring, sardines)
Live natural yoghurt
Tofu and tempeh
Seaweed (wakame, nori, arami, kelp, kombu, dulse, hijiki)

Oils and fats
Extra-virgin olive oil
Flaxseed oil
Sesame seed oil
Walnut oil
Pumpkin seed oil

Spices and flavourings
Balsamic vinegar
Chillies
Cider vinegar
Cumin
Garlic
Ginger
Hot pepper sauce
Japanese rice vinegar
Lemongrass
Paprika
Shoyu or tamari sauces rather than soy, which can contain caramel and wheat
Turmeric

Drinks
Water filters or bottles of still, low-sodium mineral water
Herbal teas of your choice
Non-dairy, calcium-fortified milk (e.g. almond, rice, sesame, soya)

3 **What to eat and drink**

Juicing

It is well worth buying a juicer whether you're on a detox or not, for the megadoses of vitamins and minerals that fresh juice can deliver in one hit. You will not get the same benefits from shop-bought 'freshly squeezed' juices; orange juice, for example, starts to lose its vitamin content seven minutes after being squeezed.

must know

Variations on a theme
Different detox diets make different dietary recommendations, particularly when it comes to protein. Carol Vorderman's plans cut all dairy, poultry and meat in the detox phase, just reintroducing them at maintenance stage. Jane Scrivner allows sheep's and goat's milk and cheese products. Some allow organic meat and poultry. Choose the one that fits your lifestyle most easily, because that's the one you are most likely to stick to.

Opposite: Squeeze a lemon or lime and strain into a glass, then add some still or fizzy water and a little fructose or honey to taste.

Have fun experimenting

You don't get all the fibre of the fruit and veg when you juice them, but the vitamin content is more than you would get otherwise because - let's face it - who would eat eight oranges in one sitting? Not many of us, but a large glass of juice might contain the juice of eight oranges.

Buy a juicer with a removeable filter so you don't have to clean the whole mechanism every time. Buy organic fruit and vegetables, and clean, peel, deseed and chop them before putting them in the juicer. Experiment with your favourite ingredients to come up with your own recipes, or try the following:

Veg-based combinations
- 3 carrots, 2 fennel stalks and ½ lemon
- 3 carrots, 2 celery stalks, a 2cm (1in) piece of fresh root ginger and ½ apple
- 3-4 carrots, 1-2 celery stalks and a small wedge of cabbage
- 1 green pepper, 1 red pepper, 3 celery stalks, ½ cucumber and 5 lettuce leaves
- 5 handfuls spinach, 1 cucumber and 2 carrots
- 1 beetroot, 2 carrots, a small handful of spinach, 2 tomatoes and a squeeze of fresh lime juice

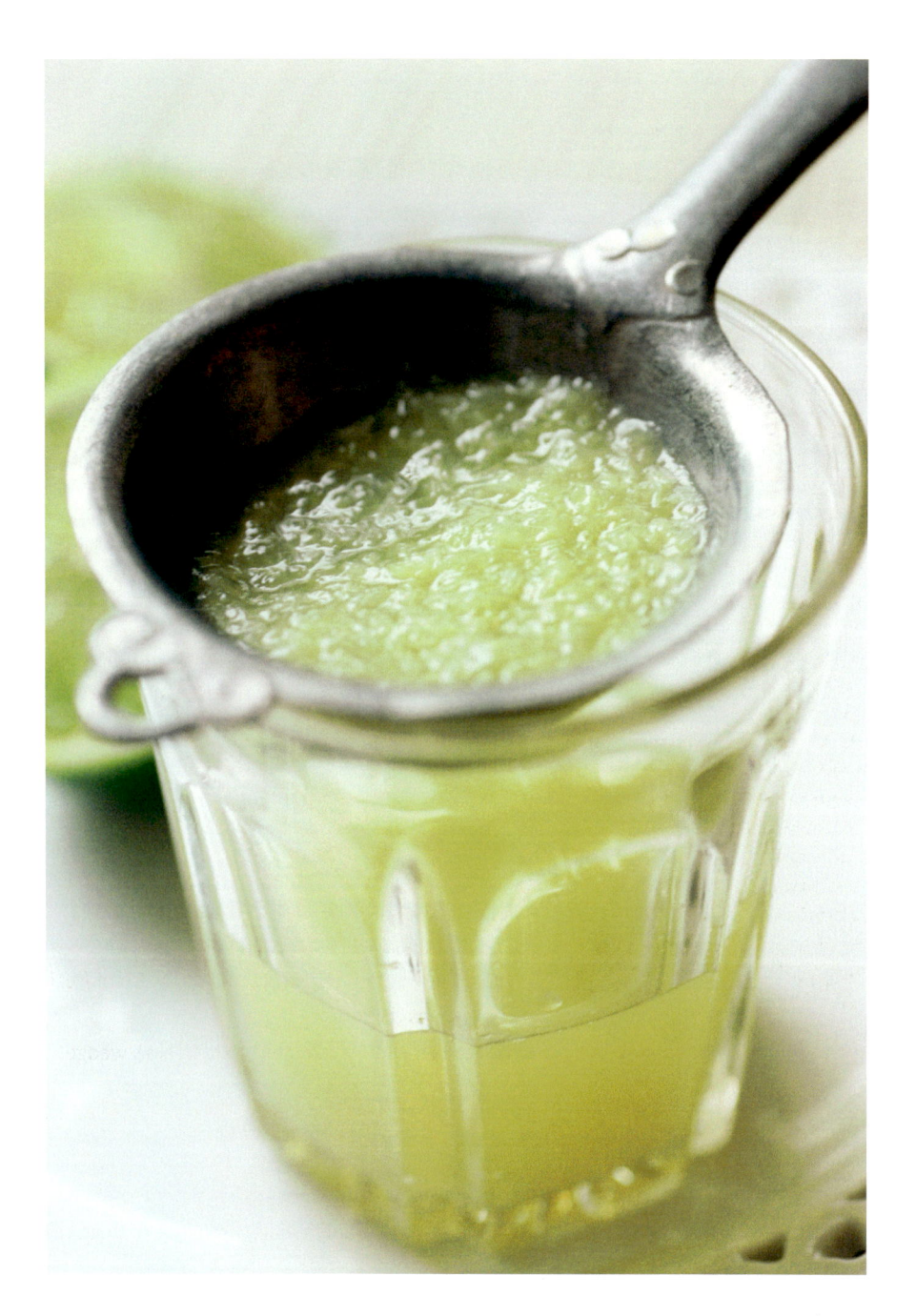

3 What to eat and drink

Try blending strawberries and bananas with some almond milk to make tasty, filling milkshakes.

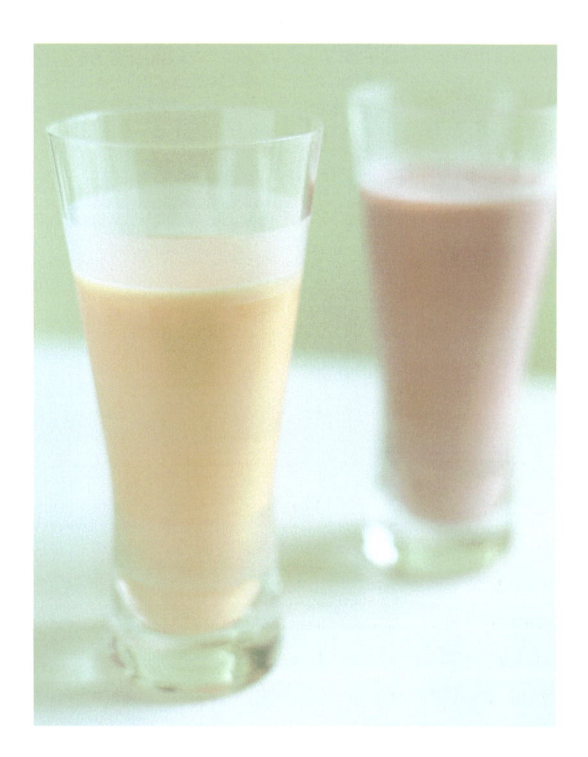

- 5 carrots, 1 apple and ½ beetroot
- ½ head of broccoli, a handful of watercress, a handful of parsley, 1 stick of celery and ½ fresh pineapple
- 4-5 carrots, ½ lemon, 1 apple, small wedge of red cabbage and a small piece of fresh root ginger
- 3 celery stalks, a handful of spinach, 2 asparagus stalks and 1 large tomato
- A large leaf each of kale and collard, a handful of parsley, 1 celery stalk, 1 carrot, ½ red pepper, 1 tomato and 1 large broccoli floret

Fruit-based combinations
- 2 apples, 2 pears and a 2cm (1in) piece of fresh root ginger

- A handful of blueberries, handful of raspberries, 1 apple and 2 nectarines
- 1 orange, 1 mango and 1 kiwi fruit
- 12 strawberries and 4-5 carrots
- A large slice of watermelon, a cup of ripe strawberries and the juice and zest of 1 lime
- 2 oranges, 4 carrots and a 2cm (1in) piece of fresh root ginger
- A large bunch of seedless grapes, 1 apple and some fresh mint leaves

Smoothies

To turn your fruit-based juice into a smoothie, just add some live natural yoghurt. Alternatively, for a fruit-based milkshake, you can add a non-dairy soya, rice or almond milk – although none of these would be allowed on a juice-based fast. Always drink your juices and shakes immediately to gain the maximum nutritional value.

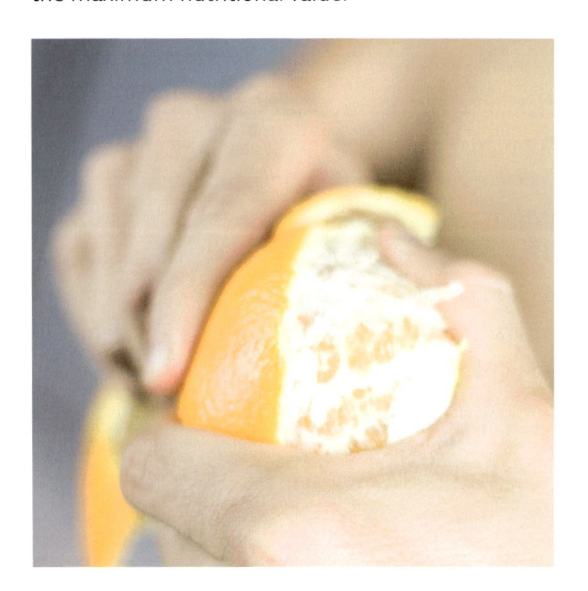

must know

Green superfoods
Wheatgrass, barley grass, alfalfa grass, blue-green algae, spirulina and chlorella have an extraordinary mixture of easily digestible nutrients, vitamins and minerals, essential fatty acids and healthy bacteria to help your system function more effectively. Buy them as powders or liquids from good health-food shops and add them to your juices for an extra blast of goodness.

Fresh orange juice can have many uses; you can marinate chicken strips in it with some garlic and shoyu sauce, or squeeze it over steamed green vegetables.

3 What to eat and drink

Time for tea

You can drink any herbal teas you fancy on a detox, but the ones featured here have special benefits to help cleanse the system. Many of the tea manufacturers now make their own 'Detox' or 'Cleansing' brands, which often contain a mixture of useful ingredients, but always buy organic teas if you can.

must know

Dandelion root coffee
Buy dandelion roots from a health food shop and allow them to dry. Place the dried roots on a baking tray in an oven preheated to 200°C, Gas Mark 6 and roast them until they are a deep brown colour. Store in a glass jar and when you are ready to use, grind them into a fine powder using a coffee mill. Add a teaspoon to a cup of boiling water, stir and then drink.

Suitable teas

Decaff coffee and tea are not recommended on a detox diet because of the methods used to extract the caffeine. The methylene chloride used in some decaffeinating processes is related to the toxic perchlorethylene used in dry cleaning. An organic solvent called ethyl acetate is also sometimes used and the product might be labelled 'naturally decaffeinated' because this chemical occurs in some fruits and in the coffee itself, but studies have shown that it is still highly toxic. Try a few of the following teas to see which you prefer – they all taste different and have specific properties, and it is a matter of personal taste which you choose.

Which tea?

• Nettle tea is a diuretic, meaning it helps your body to excrete water, so it will flush out your toxins more quickly.

• Milk thistle tea contains silymarin which makes the liver less susceptible to toxin damage and increases its production of glutathione. For more on this wonder-herb, see page 119.

• Red sorrel tea is a terrific liver and gall bladder cleanser, and a recent study has indicated that it

decreases the blood triglyceride levels (high levels are associated with heart disease and diabetes).
- Dandelion leaf tea has a diuretic action, while dandelion root coffee is an effective detox aid, stimulating the flow of bile so that more toxins are eliminated through the bowels.
- Rooibosch (or Red Bush) tea helps you to shed toxins through sweat, can relieve bloating and aid the digestive process. It is also claimed to reduce the effects of ageing, keep skin, teeth and bones healthy, and it can aid sleep.
- Chamomile tea is calming, soporific and can help to relieve mild headaches.
- Lemon balm helps with depression and anxiety.
- Spearmint and peppermint tea both aid digestion.
- Fennel tea stimulates the liver.

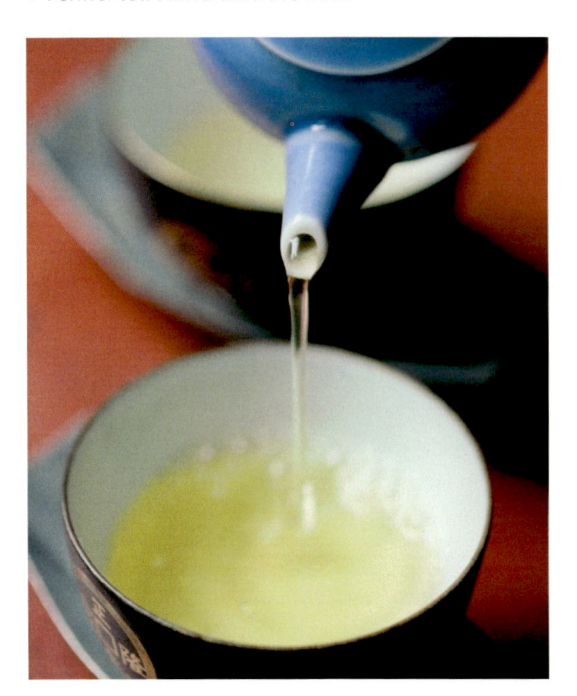

must know

Leaf tea
The herbal teabags are absolutely fine, but once you have tried making your own brew from fresh leaves there will be no going back. A big handful of mint leaves steeped in boiling water for 5 minutes makes the most delicious mint tea. Some health food shops sell herbal preparations you can use to make your own teas, and will invariably provide more taste than the powdered preparations that are used in teabags.

There is no need to forego your normal tea breaks on a detox; choose healing, nourishing teas instead of caffeine-based ones.

3 What to eat and drink

Menu plans for 7-day detox

Some diets tell you 'It's Wednesday and therefore you must have porridge' but the beauty of a week-long detox is that you can suit your own tastes. You choose what you want for breakfast, lunch, dinner and snacks, so long as you keep the ingredients varied and eat a range of different-coloured fruits and vegetables every day.

must know

Wheat substitutes
Terence Stamp produces a range of wheat-free, gluten-free breads, or you can find other varieties by reading the labels in your health food shop. Slice them carefully as wheat-free breads tend to crumble easily. Take care not to over-cook wheat-free pasta, or you can end up with a gloopy mess.

Breakfast choices

- Start-the-day cereal (see page 82)
- Oat porridge made with whole oats (not instant) and served with your choice of non-dairy milk, honey and nuts
- Millet or quinoa porridge with a dried fruit topping, served with non-dairy milk
- Compôte of mixed dried fruits soaked in orange juice and served with live yoghurt
- Non-wheat bread toasted and served with nut butter or honey
- Poached organic eggs and steamed spinach on non-wheat toast
- Fruit salad of mango, papaya and melon topped with sesame seeds

Lunch choices

- Any of the soups on pages 92–96, served with non-wheat bread to dip in
- Your selection of the salads on pages 83–91
- A Mediterranean vegetable omelette, with red onion, cherry tomatoes, courgette and peppers
- Goat's cheese salad with walnuts sprinkled on top
- Ratatouille heaped on a slice of toasted wheat-free bread

- Non-wheat pasta with steamed vegetables and a simple tomato sauce
- A baked potato filled with Greek salad – feta cheese, tomato, onion, cucumber and black olives
- Crudités with Mexican dips (see page 98)

Dinner choices
- Your choice of organic oily fish served with heaps of seasonal vegetables and a squeeze of lemon juice
- Baked salmon (see page 104) with your vegetable accompaniment of choice
- Oriental stir-fried broccoli with nuts (see page 102)
- Pasta with artichokes and olives (see page 101)
- Quinoa and wild rice pilaff (see page 103)
- Spicy cannellini bean and tomato casserole (see page 105)
- Roast vegetables with sweet potato mash (see page 106), served with fish if you like
- Masoor dhal with cauliflower (see page 107)
- Vegetable fried rice with nori (see page 108)
- Marinated vegetable kebabs (see page 109)
- A selection of roasted vegetables, including beetroot, aubergine, courgette, tomatoes and red onion, with pumpkin seeds and crumbled feta cheese on top

Desserts
- Any kind of fresh fruit salad
- Pomegranate ice (see page 110)
- Orange and date salad (see page 111)
- Blueberry salad (see page 111)
- Rice pudding made with non-dairy milk
- Crumbles made with oat and crushed nut toppings

must know

Sandwich fillings
Make sandwiches that will make your non-detoxing friends drool.
- Hummus, avocado and grated carrot
- Smoked tofu, grated roast beetroot and sprouting seeds
- Sliced grilled courgette, mozzarella and sun-blush tomatoes
- Cold roast vegetables on mixed salad leaves
- Stoned black olives mashed into a tapenade paste, slices of plum tomato and artichoke heart

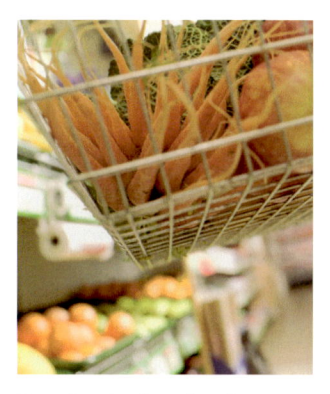

Try to buy local produce in season from farmers' markets and small greengrocers to get the freshest possible food.

3 What to eat and drink

must know

Eating out
It's not easy to eat in restaurants when you are detoxing, as you'll have to quiz waiters endlessly about cooking methods and added ingredients. Even vegetarian restaurants can rely heavily on wheat and cheese. Choose a large salad with grilled fish (if you are having fish on your detox) – or leave eating out for the post-detox period.

When making fruit salad, mix sweet and tart flavours and two or three different textures.

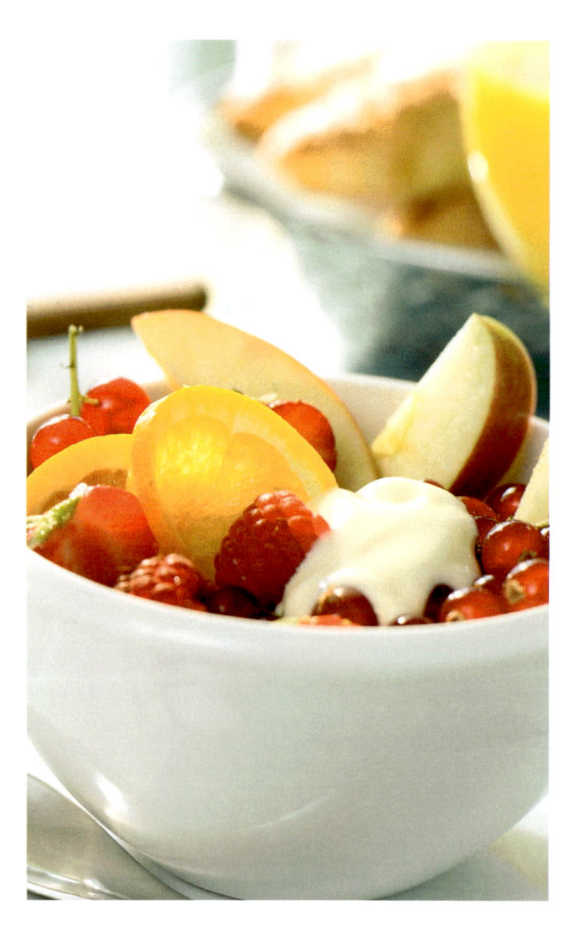

Detox snacks
- Rice cakes (unsalted, plain or sesame seed), oatcakes or non-wheat bread with hummus, tahini, guacamole, goat's cheese, nut butter or honey
- Some cherry tomatoes with a few chunks of goat's cheese
- Half an avocado sprinkled with olive oil and balsamic vinegar
- Mixed nuts and seeds (health food shops have lots of nutritious mixtures)

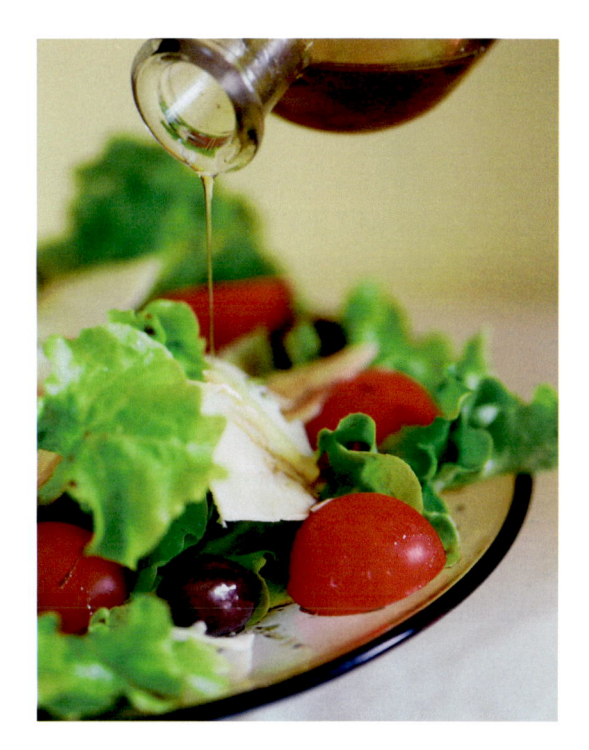

Avoid shop-bought salad dressing which can have a lot of additives. Drizzle over some good oil with vinegar or lemon juice to taste.

want to know more?

• Carol Vorderman's books (see page 190) are full of inspiring detox recipes and she provides a 28-day menu plan in *Detox for Life*.
• For supplements to take during a detox, see pages 116–121.

weblinks

• For information on organic foods, go to: www.soilassociation.org
• You can enter a plant food and find out about the pesticides used on it and the health risks associated with them on: www.foodnews.org/tools.php
• To find out more about drinking water, see the Drinking Water Inspectorate's website: www.dwi.org.gov.uk
• For water filters, see: www.kombuchatea.co.uk

• Raw vegetable crudités served with tahini, hummus or guacamole
• Some raisins or other dried fruits
• Any fresh fruit – melon, grapes, apple, pear, satsuma
• A fresh juice, smoothie or non-dairy milk shake

Post-detox dinners

• Any detox salads or vegetable dishes served with grilled organic meat, fish or chicken
• Pepper steak with two salads (see page 113)
• Chicken with chickpeas, olives and lemon (see page 112)
• Oriental stir-fries with fish or chicken
• All kinds of curry dishes

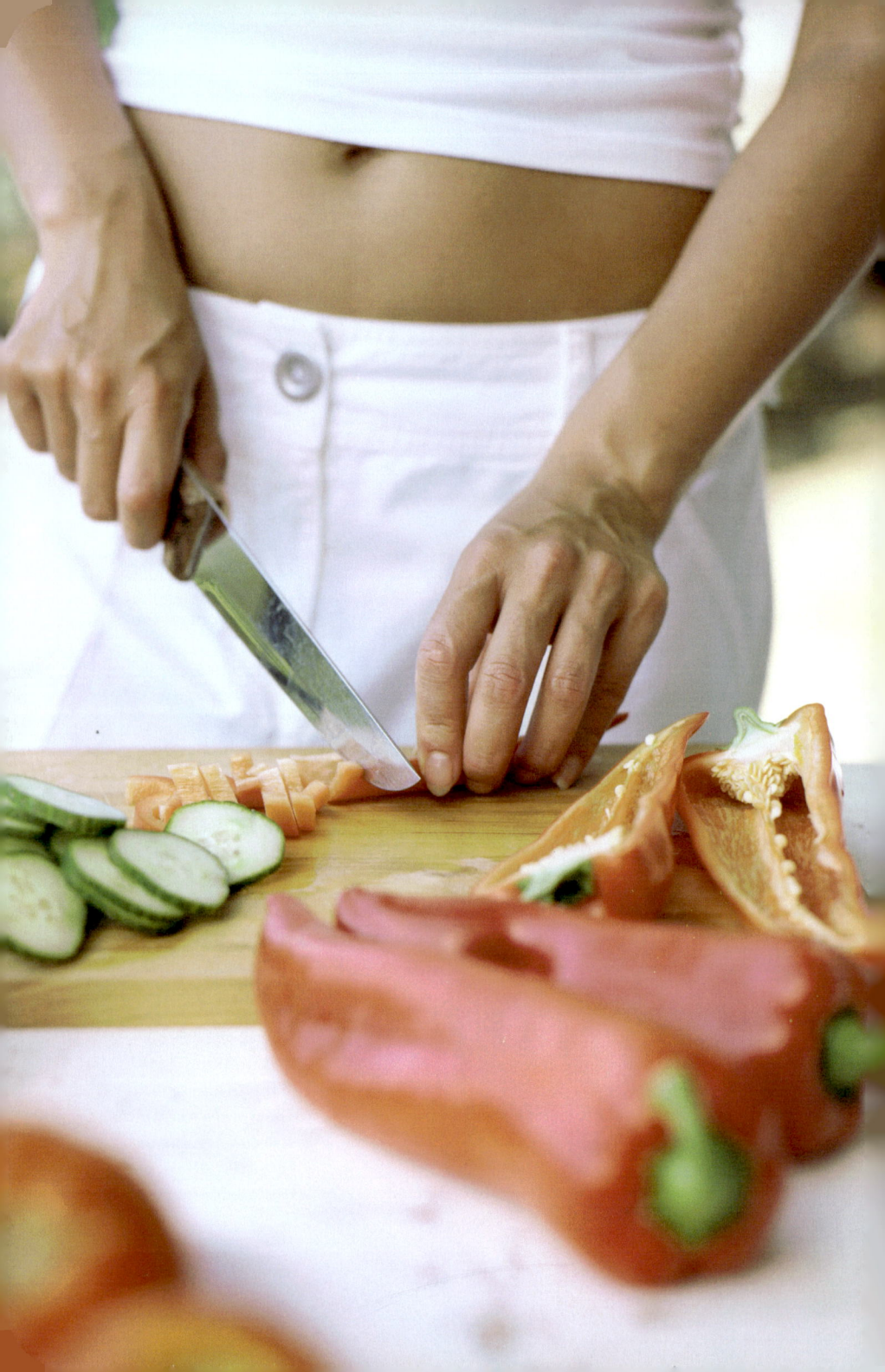

4 Detox recipes

Don't worry – it's not all broccoli and brown rice. Detox food should be colourful, tasty and full of different textures and flavours to make it interesting and satisfying to eat. The recipes featured in this chapter all serve one, unless otherwise indicated, and they are presented so that if you are on a strict vegan detox, you can omit the fish, cheese or yoghurt additions.

4 Detox recipes

Start-the-day cereal

(serves 1) This provides a good dose of fibre, B vitamins, iron, magnesium, zinc, omega-3 and omega-6 fatty acids from the seeds, protein and minerals from the nuts, and vitamin C from the fruit. Adjust the quantities according to appetite and preference.

Ingredients

4-5 dsp whole oat flakes
1-2 dsp sunflower seeds
1-2 dsp pumpkin seeds
4-5 Brazil nuts *or* 6-8 other unsalted nuts of your choice
½ dessertspoon organic dried fruit (this may not be necessary if your fresh fruit is sweet enough)
non-dairy soya, almond or rice milk
fresh fruit in season, e.g. strawberries, raspberries, chopped mango, peach, pear or apple, gooseberries, blueberries.

The oat flakes are easiest to digest if you soak them in the milk for a couple of hours (or leave them overnight in the fridge). Toasting in a hot oven or dry-frying brings out the flavour of the sunflower and pumpkins seeds. But if you're in a hurry, as most of us are in the morning, you can just place all the ingredients in a bowl and eat.

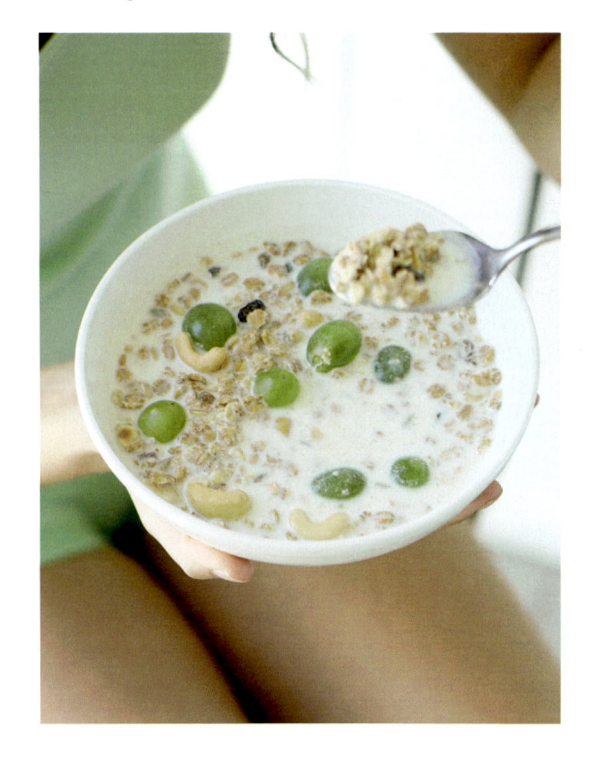

Avocado and tomato salad with shallots

(serves 1) You can add mozzarella cheese to this recipe if you wish, for a classic Italian *tricolore* salad.

Put the finely chopped shallot in a small bowl or container, such as an egg cup, with the balsamic vinegar while you prepare the salad.

Arrange the sliced tomatoes on one side of a plate. Cut the avocado into halves and remove the stone; cut through the flesh to the skin but not through the skin itself. Starting at the pointed end, peel the skin away with your fingers; if the avocado is ripe enough, this should be easy. Arrange the avocado slices on the other half of the plate.

Carefully, using a teaspoon, arrange the chopped shallot in a fine line between the two halves, leaving any excess vinegar behind. Drizzle olive oil over the salad, grind some black pepper over everything and put a little salt on the tomatoes. Serve immediately.

Ingredients

1 large shallot *or* 2 smaller ones, peeled and finely chopped
2 tsp balsamic vinegar
3 medium tomatoes, sliced
1 ripe avocado
olive oil
salt and black pepper

4 Detox recipes

Warm asparagus and courgette salad

(*serves 1*) Asparagus is high in glutathione, which helps your liver to function effectively, while courgettes are a good source of potassium, betacarotene and vitamin C.

Ingredients

6-10 hazelnuts
250g (8oz) bunch of asparagus
a large handful of salad leaves
½ large courgette
salt and black pepper

For the dressing:
½ tsp Dijon mustard
½ tsp clear honey
juice of ½ small lemon
1 tsp olive oil

Chop the hazelnuts and then dry-roast them in a non-stick pan; when they start to smell toasted, remove the pan from the heat.

Fill a large pan with water and put it on to boil. Trim the woody ends from the asparagus and then discard them (they can go towards vegetable stock if you wish). Cut the remaining stems halfway along and put the thicker, lower halves into the boiling water for 3 minutes. Now add the rest of the asparagus to the pan of boiling water and cook for 2 minutes.

Make the dressing: whisk the mustard, honey, lemon juice and olive oil together until smooth. Arrange the salad leaves on a plate.

Meanwhile, make long strips of courgette with a potato peeler; discard any which are entirely peel and also get rid of the rather seedy core. Add the strips to the asparagus and cook for a further minute.

Drain and allow to cool briefly until the asparagus can be handled, and then arrange both the asparagus pieces and the courgette strips on top of the salad leaves. Whisk the dressing once more and drizzle it over everything, season with salt and black pepper and scatter the hazelnuts on top. Serve immediately.

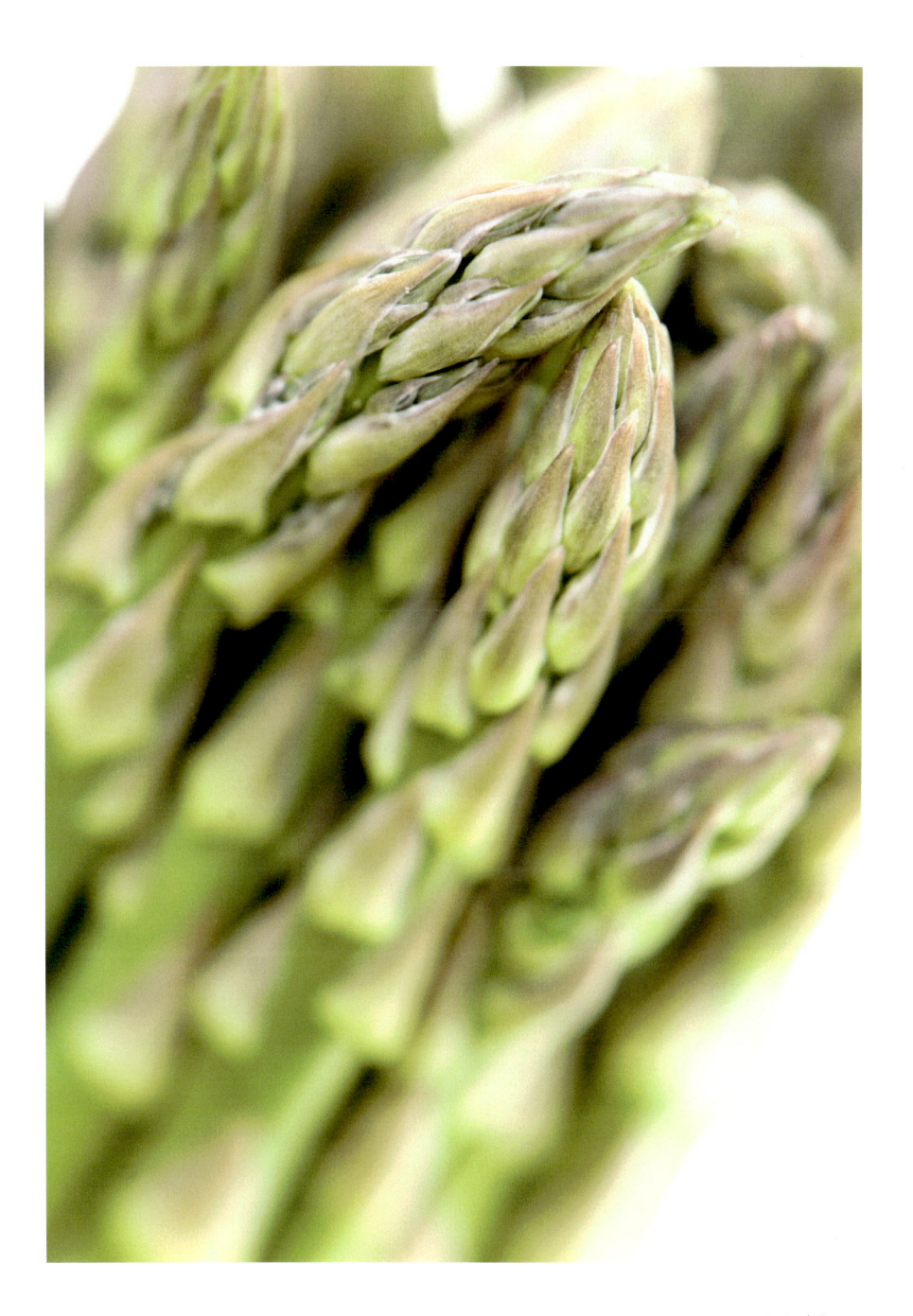

4 Detox recipes

Detox 'coleslaw' with seeds

(serves 2) You might well decide to make a larger batch of this delicious salad and save some for later, but do not add the seeds until you are ready to serve it.

Ingredients

75g (3oz) white cabbage, finely shredded
2 carrots, grated
½ yellow pepper, seeded and finely chopped
1 small red onion, finely chopped
6 black olives, chopped
1 tsp pumpkin seeds
1 tsp sunflower seeds

For the dressing:
1 tbsp apple juice
1 tsp olive oil
½ tsp Dijon mustard
1 tsp lemon juice
salt and black pepper

Put the cabbage, carrots, yellow pepper, onions and olives in a large bowl.

Put all the dressing ingredients in a jar, make sure the lid is screwed on tightly, and shake well. Taste and adjust the seasoning, then pour over the vegetables and stir well.

Dry-roast the pumpkin and sunflower seeds in a dry frying pan, stirring them so they don't catch too much. Remove the pan from the heat when they begin to colour.

Put the coleslaw on a serving plate and scatter the seeds on top. Serve immediately.

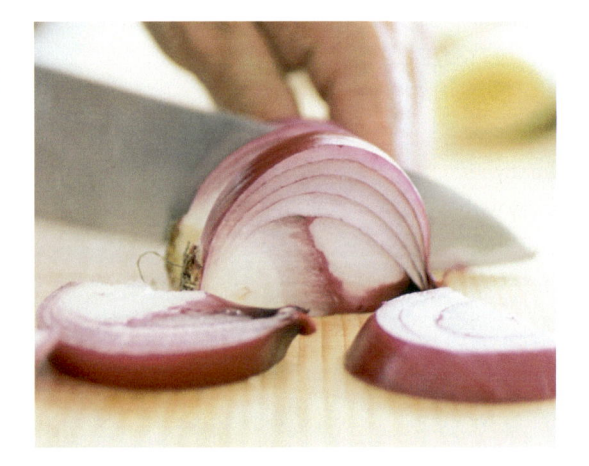

Lentil and roast pepper salad

(serves 1) If you are eating cheese on your detox, crumble some goat's cheese or feta over the top of this delicious salad.

Preheat the oven to 200°C/Gas Mark 6. Rub the outside of each pepper half with olive oil and put them, cut side down, in an ovenproof dish. Roast them in the oven for 15–20 minutes until the skins begin to blister and darken. Set aside until just cool enough to handle.

Meanwhile, put the lentils into a pan of boiling water and cook until soft; how long this takes will depend on their age, but it should be approximately the same time as the peppers – about 20 minutes.

Make the dressing: whisk the balsamic vinegar (or lemon juice), olive oil and mustard together. Add a little salt and black pepper to taste, and whisk again.

Drain the lentils and put them in a large bowl; pour most of the dressing over them while they are warm, add the onion and stir thoroughly.

Gently remove the skin from the peppers, easing it away with a knife if necessary, and cut the flesh into strips. Add to the lentils with the red onion, mixing them in gently. Arrange the salad leaves on a plate, drizzle the remaining dressing over them and put the lentils and peppers in the middle. Garnish with flat-leaved parsley and serve immediately.

Ingredients

1 large red pepper, halved and seeded
a little olive oil
60g (2oz) green lentils, e.g. Le Puy, rinsed well
½ small red onion, chopped
salad leaves
flat-leaved parsley, to garnish

For the dressing:

2 tsp balsamic vinegar (or lemon juice)
1 tsp olive oil
¼ tsp Dijon mustard
salt and black pepper

4 Detox recipes

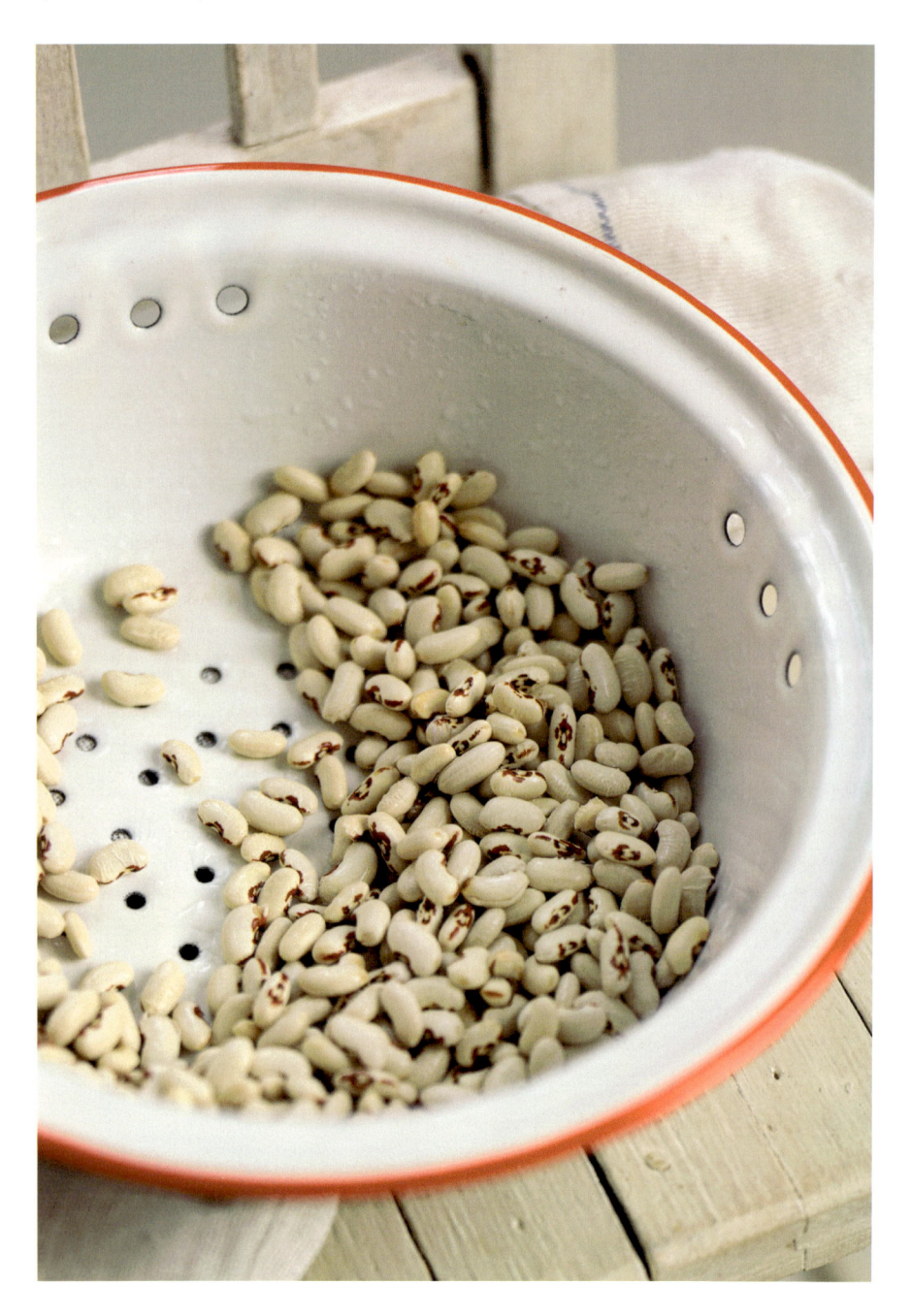

Bean salad with herbs and wild leaves

(*serves 1*) This makes a very filling dish for lunch on days when you are starving. The beans and chickpeas are a great source of protein, fibre and minerals.

Soak the haricots, black-eye beans and chickpeas overnight, keeping the haricots separate. Drain and rinse all of them, and put the haricots into a small pan with fresh water. Bring to the boil, then simmer gently. When they are beginning to soften, add the chickpeas and continue cooking until tender.

Put the black-eye beans in another pan, cover with fresh water and boil for 10 minutes, then reduce the heat and simmer until tender.

Meanwhile, make the dressing. Mix the lemon juice, olive oil, black pepper, mustard and honey in a jar, close it tightly and then shake well.

Drain the cooked beans and rinse with fresh water. Put all the beans in a bowl and add half the dressing. Then add the chopped onion, olives and tomatoes, and mix well. Check the seasoning.

Mix the salad leaves and dandelion greens in another bowl and pour the other half of the dressing over them. Toss and then arrange on a plate, leaving a gap in the middle for the beans. Add the beans and serve immediately.

Ingredients

20g ($^2/_3$oz) dried haricot beans
20g ($^2/_3$oz) dried black-eye beans
40g (1$^1/_2$oz) dried chickpeas
1 small red onion, chopped
6 olives, chopped
6 cherry tomatoes, chopped
salad leaves, e.g. rocket, coriander and flat-leaved parsley
a handful of small dandelion leaves
salt and black pepper

For the dressing:
1 tbsp lemon juice
2 tsp olive oil
black pepper
$^1/_2$ tsp wholegrain mustard
$^1/_2$ tsp clear honey

4 Detox recipes

Kiwi, avocado and spring onion salad

(*serves 1*) You might think that this sounds like an odd mixture, but you will be converted when you try it. Kiwis are one of the best fruit sources of vitamin C.

Ingredients

1 kiwi fruit
3 spring onions
1 ripe avocado
salad leaves

For the dressing:
a squeeze of lime juice
1 tsp olive oil
a dab of honey (about ½ teaspoon, or to taste)
salt and black pepper

Peel the kiwi fruit, cut into slices and then cut each slice into four. Finely chop the spring onions, and put them, with the kiwi, into a bowl.

Make the dressing. Put the lime juice, olive oil and honey in a screwtop jar with lots of freshly ground black pepper. Seal the jar and shake it well, then taste, adding a little salt if wished. Pour over the kiwi and spring onions and leave for 30 minutes for the flavours to develop.

Cut the avocado in half and remove the stone; peel and then chop the flesh into chunks. Add these to the bowl containing the kiwi and spring onions, and stir very gently to coat the pieces in the dressing.

Arrange the salad leaves on a plate and arrange the kiwi, spring onion and avocado in the middle. Serve the salad immediately.

Tomato, onion and herb salad

(serves 1) Prepare this in advance and leave to allow the flavours to mingle. Tomatoes sold on the vine often taste best.

Rinse the red onion in cold water, then soak for 10 minutes and chop coarsely – you need slightly less onion than tomatoes. Mix the chopped onion with the tomatoes in a large bowl, add the olive oil and a good grinding of black pepper, and stir well. Then cover the bowl with clingfilm and refrigerate for at least 1 hour.

Strip the leaves from the stems of the coriander and flat-leaved parsley, chop them roughly and add to the onion and tomato mixture. Stir well and add a little more olive oil if you like. Check the seasoning and serve immediately.

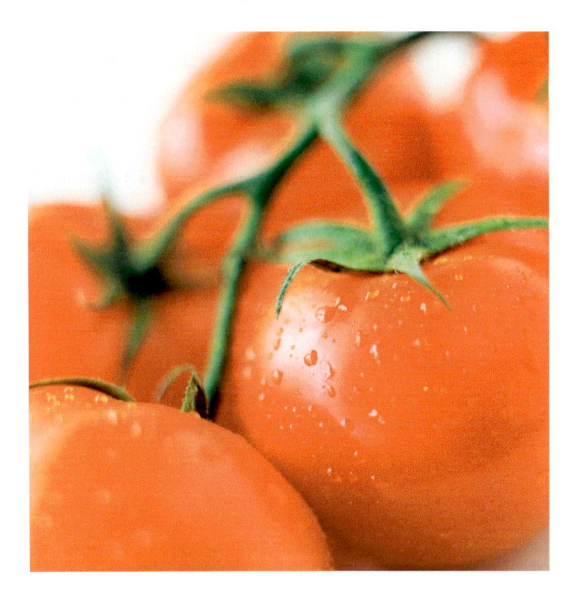

Ingredients

1 red onion, peeled and halved
3 medium tomatoes, seeded and chopped
1 tbsp olive oil
a large handful of coriander leaves
a large handful of flat-leaved parsley
salt and black pepper

4 Detox recipes

Light spinach, parsley, lemon and garlic soup

(serves 2) Make your own vegetable stock rather than using a stock cube, which could contain sugar, salt and artificial flavours and preservatives. You can buy organic bouillon powder.

Ingredients

1 small onion, chopped
1 tsp olive oil
2 garlic cloves, chopped
a large handful of fresh parsley, chopped
225g (8oz) fresh spinach, chopped
400ml (14fl oz) vegetable stock *or* water
juice of ½ lemon
salt and black pepper
grated nutmeg (optional)
sprigs of parsley, to garnish

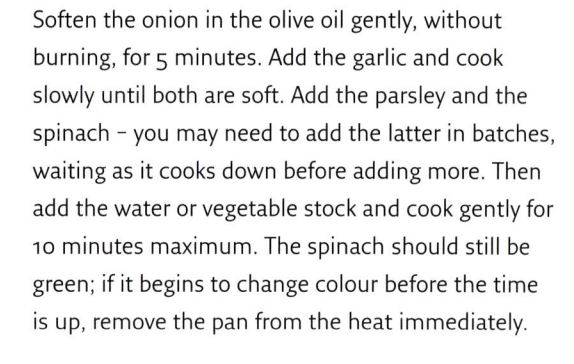

Soften the onion in the olive oil gently, without burning, for 5 minutes. Add the garlic and cook slowly until both are soft. Add the parsley and the spinach – you may need to add the latter in batches, waiting as it cooks down before adding more. Then add the water or vegetable stock and cook gently for 10 minutes maximum. The spinach should still be green; if it begins to change colour before the time is up, remove the pan from the heat immediately.

Stir in the lemon juice and allow the soup to cool a little. Blend, adjusting the consistency if wished by adding a little more liquid. Check the seasoning, reheat gently and add a little grated nutmeg (optional). Serve garnished with parsley.

Vegetable stock

To make your own vegetable stock, slice 1 onion, 2 leeks, 1 fennel bulb and 2 carrots. Place in a large saucepan with some fresh parsley sprigs, coriander seeds, bay leaves and thyme, cover with water and simmer for 45 minutes, then strain.

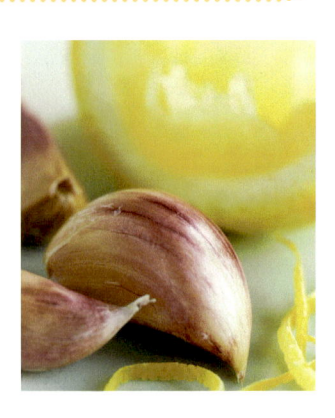

Carrot and lentil soup

(*Serves 2*) The old wives' tale is true – carrots can help you to see in the dark. They can also boost your immune system, make your skin healthier and protect against lung cancer.

Warm the oil in a heavy pan, add the chopped red onion and cook gently, allowing it to brown a little, for 5 minutes. Add the carrots, stir well, and cook for 2 minutes before adding the stock or water and the lentils. Cook for 20 minutes and then add the orange or mandarin juice.

Remove the thyme leaves from the sprigs and drop them into the soup (reserve some for later). Cook for 5 minutes and add some black pepper. Remove from the heat, allow to cool a little and then blend, adding more liquid if you prefer a thinner soup. Reheat gently, check the seasoning and serve, garnished with the reserved thyme leaves.

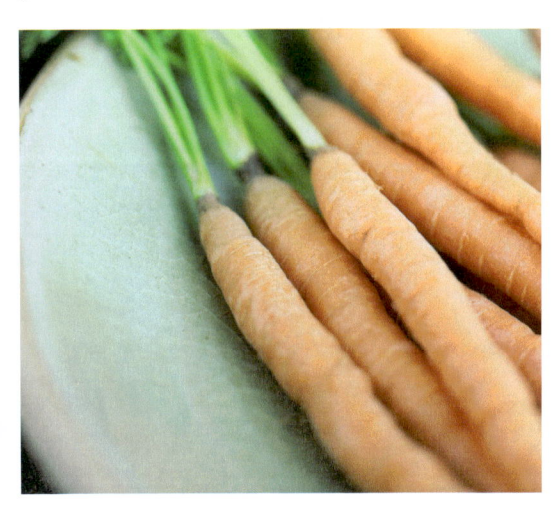

Ingredients

1 tsp olive oil
1 small red onion, chopped
200g (7oz) carrots, chopped
650ml (1 pint 2fl oz) vegetable stock or water
30g (1oz) green lentils, picked over and rinsed
juice of ½ small orange *or* 1 mandarin
a few sprigs of fresh thyme
salt and black pepper

4 Detox recipes

Sweetcorn soup

(serves 2) Sweetcorn provides fibre, folic acid and antioxidants. You can make this soup spicier if you like, but be warned – it's very moreish! This quantity of cayenne produces quite an oomph, but more can be added. If you like hot flavours, then a few flakes of dried red chilli can also be scattered on top as a garnish.

Ingredients

1 medium onion, chopped
1 tsp olive oil
pinch of cayenne pepper, to taste
1 x 200g (7oz) can organic sweetcorn, drained
600 ml (1 pint) vegetable stock *or* water
salt and black pepper

Soften the onion in the olive oil gently in a pan with a lid; don't let it burn but allow it to colour a little. When the onion is soft, add the cayenne pepper and stir thoroughly. Add the sweetcorn and the stock or water. Cover and cook gently for 25 minutes – the liquid will reduce quite a lot.

Blend the soup thoroughly in a food processor or blender and check the consistency, adding another 100 ml (3½ fl oz) liquid if wished. Reheat gently and season to taste before serving.

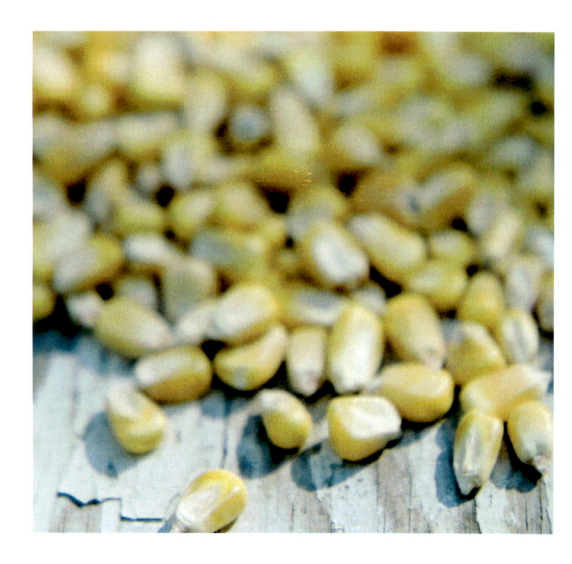

Chickpea, courgette and tomato soup

(serves 2) Chickpeas contain a particular kind of fibre that helps the beneficial bacteria in the intestine to do their work. Some nutritionists also claim they have antidepressant qualities.

Soak the chickpeas overnight. Rinse and drain them, put into fresh water and boil for 10 minutes, removing any froth that forms. Drain and rinse.

Warm the olive oil in a large saucepan with a lid. Add the onion and cook gently until translucent, then add the garlic and cook for 2 minutes, stirring to ensure that nothing burns. Add the courgettes and stir for 1–2 minutes.

Stir in the chickpeas, tomatoes and enough liquid to cover everything – filling the empty tomato can will make sure that you get all the tomato juice. Add the dried herbs and then cook gently until the chickpeas are tender, about 25 minutes, depending on how fresh they are. Serve the soup in bowls, garnished with a few fresh herb leaves.

Ingredients

60g (2oz) dried chickpeas
1 tsp olive oil
1 onion, chopped
2 garlic cloves, finely chopped
2 courgettes (1 green and 1 yellow, if possible), chopped into slices and quarter slices
1 x 200g (7oz) can organic chopped tomatoes
water *or* vegetable stock
½ tsp dried Italian herb mix
fresh herbs, e.g. basil, marjoram, oregano, to garnish

Chilled beetroot soup

(serves 2) Medics researching blood cholesterol levels think beetroot may help the liver to remove the harmful kind of cholesterol from the blood, so you will be doing your guests a favour. This soup is served cold but it is also good hot. Simply reheat it after blending and don't push it through the sieve.

Ingredients

1 tsp olive oil
½ small onion, chopped
1 garlic clove, chopped
3 raw beetroot
½ tsp ground cumin
200-300g (7-10oz) canned chopped organic tomatoes
300ml (½ pint) water *or* vegetable stock
salt and black pepper
live yoghurt (optional)

Heat the oil in a saucepan, add the onion and garlic and cook gently for about 5 minutes until softened.

Prepare the beetroot: trim and peel them quickly, chop into slices, cut the slices into quarters and add them to the pan – doing this swiftly will retain more juice. Cook for 5 minutes, then stir in the cumin and tomatoes with the water or stock. Simmer gently until the beetroot is just tender, probably about 20 minutes. If the liquid looks as though it is going down rather fast, add a little more.

Blend in a liquidizer and season to taste with salt and pepper. Push the soup through a sieve into 2 serving bowls using a wooden spoon. When you've worked all the juice through, scrape the underside of the sieve into the bowls but discard any beetroot and tomato actually remaining in it.

Put the bowls of soup in the fridge and chill for at least 2 hours. Serve with a swirl of live yoghurt if wished. Adding a couple of ice cubes looks refreshing (and keeps it cold).

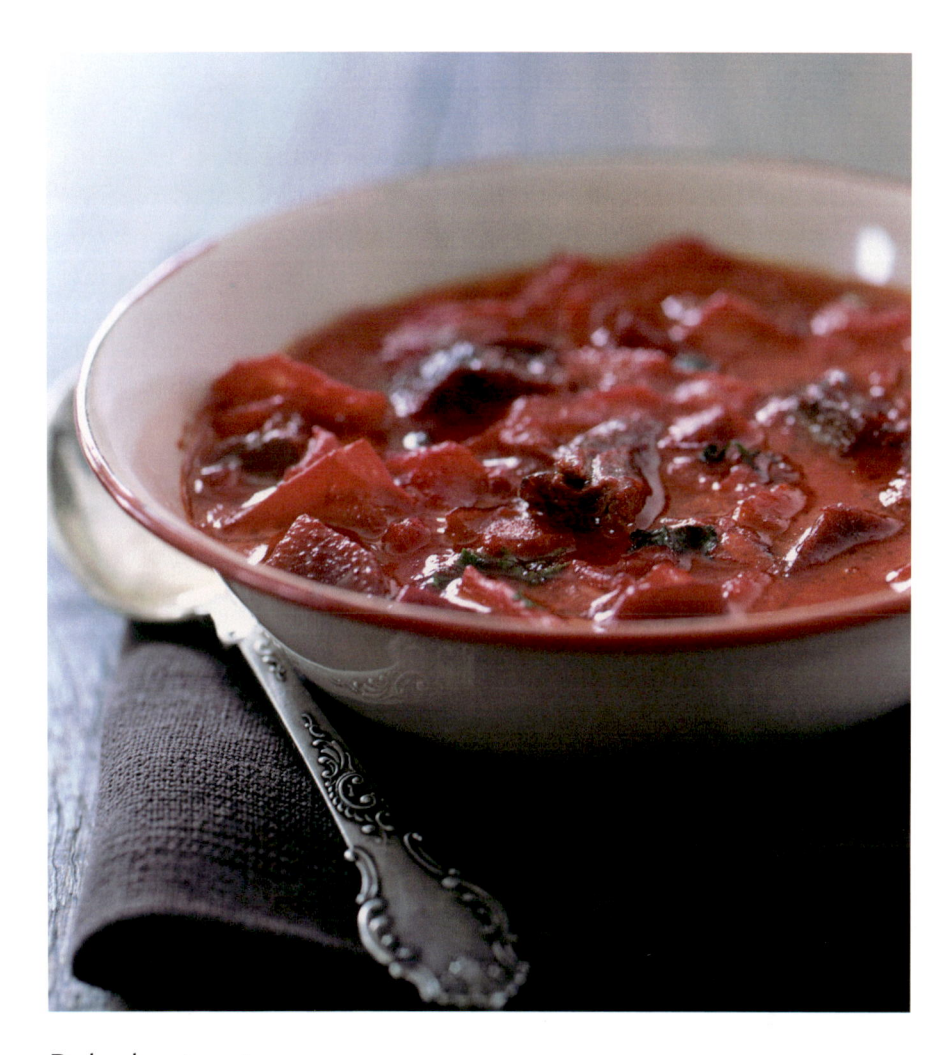

Ruby beetroot

Don't let the beetroot overcook. If it is cooked in a soup for too long, the deep ruby colour turns to a less attractive brown – so be sure to catch it in time. Around 30 minutes is the maximum cooking time.

# 4 Detox recipes

Crudités with Mexican dips

(serves 1, generously, or 2) Make the salsa and red chilli bean dips first and set aside for the flavours to mingle. You can also make the guacamole in advance but it may discolour slightly.

Ingredients

Use some of the following: spring onions; carrots, peppers and cucumber; celery sticks; chicory, cos or radicchio; cherry tomatoes; button mushrooms; cauliflower florets; radishes

Red chilli bean dip
50g (2oz) dried kidney beans
100g (3½oz) canned chopped tomatoes
1 garlic clove, chopped
pinch of chilli powder
squeeze of lemon juice
salt and black pepper

Guacamole:
1 ripe avocado, peeled and stoned
2 spring onions, chopped
1 red chilli, chopped
1 small tomato, seeded and finely chopped
squeeze of lemon juice
1 garlic clove, crushed

To make the red chilli bean dip: soak the beans overnight, then drain, rinse and put them in a pan. Cover with fresh water and boil for 15 minutes. Drain again and transfer to a clean pan. Add the tomatoes, garlic and chilli powder and simmer gently until the beans are soft, about 20 minutes. If they show signs of sticking, add a little more liquid. Cool slightly, then blend to a paste. Add the lemon juice, blend again and check the seasoning. Decant into a serving bowl and allow to cool completely. Before serving, grind black pepper over the top.

To make the guacamole: mash the avocado flesh roughly with a fork. Add the rest of the ingredients and mash everything together well; check the taste and add a little black pepper. Decant into a serving bowl. If you need to store this dip, cover it and place it in the fridge – letting the avocado stone sit in it during storage is supposed to stop it discolouring, but if you only keep it a short while and cover it well this should not be a problem.

Serve the dips surrounded by a selection of raw vegetables.

Salsa

To make the salsa: dip the tomatoes briefly in boiling water – the skins should split, making it easier to peel them. Squeeze out the seeds and chop the flesh, then put in a serving bowl. Stir in the red onion and basil. Pour a little olive oil and balsamic vinegar over the top and leave for several hours to let the flavours develop.

Ingredients

6 ripe plum tomatoes
½ red onion, finely chopped
a handful of fresh basil leaves, torn
splash of olive oil and balsamic vinegar

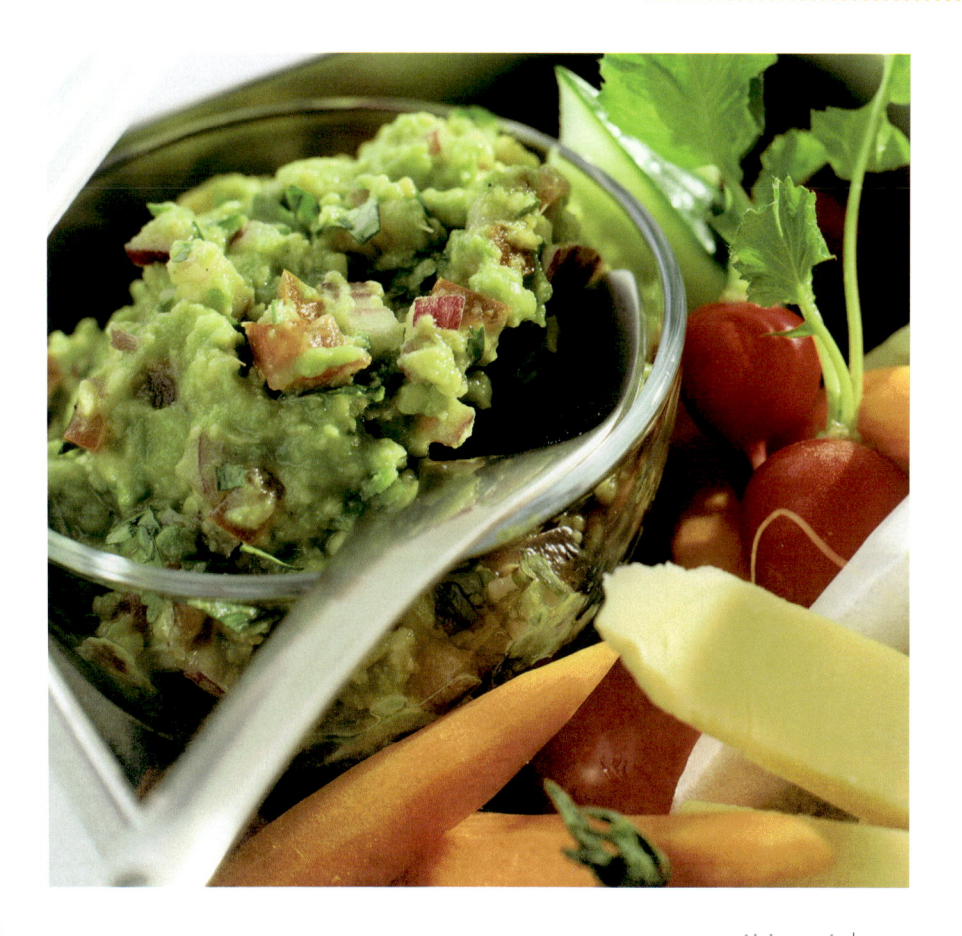

4 Detox recipes

Pasta a picchi pacchi

(serves 1) This traditional Sicilian pasta sauce is served raw and cold on hot pasta, and is simply delicious. You can use any pasta of your choice – dried (as below) or fresh.

Ingredients

250g (8oz) fresh plum tomatoes, peeled and chopped
1 tbsp olive oil
15g ($\frac{1}{2}$oz) blanched almonds, crushed
1 garlic clove, crushed
a handful of fresh basil, pounded with a mortar and pestle
small pinch of chopped chilli (optional)
75g (3oz) wheat-free spaghetti

Put all the ingredients except the spaghetti in a bowl. Cover and leave for at least 1 hour at room temperature for the flavours to mingle.

Cook the spaghetti in a large pan of boiling water for about 6–8 minutes, or according to the packet instructions. Drain and serve with the raw sauce.

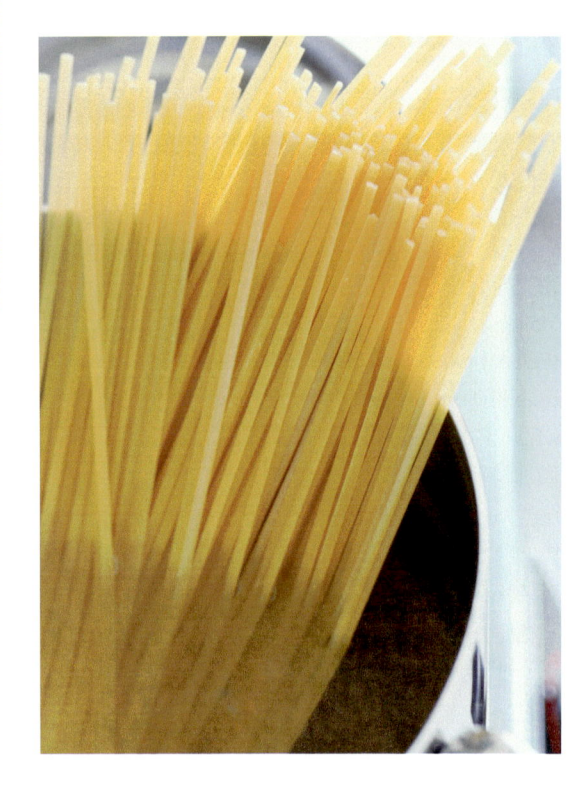

Pasta with artichokes and olives

(*serves 1*) Artichokes contain flavonoids that protect liver cells and aid the secretion of bile which helps us to digest fats. All in all, they are a class A detox food.

Bring a pan of water to a rolling boil, then add the pasta. Cook for about 6–8 minutes, or according to the instructions on the packet.

When the pasta is nearly done, warm the olive oil in a frying pan and add the garlic. When it begins to colour, stir in the chopped artichokes and olives and warm them through.

Drain the pasta, then return it to the pan, and add the artichokes, olives and garlic from the frying pan. Season with salt and black pepper, and stir in the chopped parsley. Serve immediately.

Seasonal artichokes

Make the most of fresh artichokes in season. Wash them, removing any discoloured or damaged leaves, then boil until an outside leaf comes away easily when pulled – this takes about 30 minutes for a large artichoke. Drain upside-down, then turn it right-side up and serve. Pull the leaves away and dip the bottom part of each one into vinaigrette; scrape off the base with your teeth. When you get down to the middle, remove the spiky 'choke' by slicing it off or pulling it away with a spoon. Then eat the base with a knife and fork.

Ingredients

75g (3oz) wheat-free pasta, preferably spaghetti or penne (dry weight)
1 tsp olive oil
1 garlic clove, chopped
5 pieces of artichoke from a jar of artichokes in olive oil, drained and chopped
6 olives, chopped
a handful of flat-leaved parsley, roughly chopped
salt and black pepper

4 Detox recipes

Oriental stir-fried broccoli with nuts

(*serves 1*) If you are flicking through this section, trying to decide which recipe to make, stop here. This dish is a knock-out mixture of textures, flavours, colours and healthy nutrients.

Ingredients

200g (7oz) purple sprouting broccoli
10g (⅓oz) sesame seeds
10g (⅓oz) cashew nuts
1 tsp sesame oil
4 radishes, trimmed and sliced diagonally
4 large spring onions, trimmed and sliced diagonally
½ red pepper, seeded and chopped
½ yellow pepper, seeded and chopped
2.5cm (1in) fresh root ginger, peeled and finely chopped
½ red chilli, seeded and finely chopped (or more, to taste)
1 garlic clove, finely chopped
dash of shoyu or light soy sauce
salt and black pepper

Cut the broccoli florets, with their thinner stalks attached, off the woody stems and save some of the smaller leaves. Discard the thick stalks and any particularly large and tough-looking leaves.

Dry-roast the sesame seeds and cashew nuts in a dry frying pan. When they suddenly begin to smell really toasted and colour up, remove the pan from the heat and set aside.

Heat the sesame oil in a non-stick wok, and add the radishes, spring onions and peppers when it is really hot. Stir-fry for 2 minutes, then add the ginger, chilli and garlic. When the peppers begin to soften, add the broccoli and stir-fry everything for a few more minutes. Add a dash of shoyu or light soy sauce and continue cooking until the broccoli is just beginning to soften – it should retain some crunch. Add the toasted cashews and sesame seeds and stir well. Check the seasoning, and serve immediately.

Quinoa and wild rice pilaff

(serves 1) Quinoa (pronounced 'keenwa') is easy to cook and is a complete protein, containing all the amino acids that are essential for good health (see page 51).

Put the wild rice in about 150ml (¼ pint) water, bring to the boil and simmer until cooked, about 40–50 minutes. Drain and set aside.

Warm the oil in a heavy-based pan with a lid, and add the onion. When it begins to soften, add the cardamom, cinnamon and black pepper. Add the quinoa and stir for 2–3 minutes. Add 200ml (7fl oz) water and bring to the boil, then reduce the heat, cover and cook, undisturbed, for 10 minutes.

Add the pine nuts and check the liquid, adding some more if necessary, and stir. Cook, covered, for 3 minutes, then check again and add the apricots. Stir in the cooked rice and cook, uncovered, until all the liquid has been absorbed – you will need to stir continuously to prevent it sticking. Check the seasoning, adding harissa or chilli sauce if liked. Serve, garnished with mint leaves.

Ingredients

10g (⅓oz) wild rice
350–500ml (12–16fl oz) water
1 tsp rapeseed oil
1 small red onion, chopped
2 cardamom pods, crushed
a small pinch of cinnamon
black pepper
40g (1½oz) quinoa
20 pine nuts
2 dried apricots, chopped
harissa or chilli sauce (optional)
small mint leaves, to garnish (optional)

Wild rice

This is actually the seed of a grass unrelated to ordinary rice, and has a delicious, almost smoky flavour. It also takes longer to cook but can be cooked in advance, even up to a day beforehand. Keep cooked wild rice covered in the fridge if it is going to be some time before you use it.

4 Detox recipes

Baked salmon

(serves 1) This would go well with Quinoa and Wild Rice Pilaff (see page 103), Vegetable Fried Rice with Nori (see page 108), or with Oriental Stir-fried Broccoli with Nuts (see page 102). Alternatively, for a quick and easy supper after work, roast some vegetables in the oven while the salmon is baking, or serve the salmon with a large mixed salad in a lemony dressing.

Ingredients

1 stick lemongrass, chopped into a few large pieces
1 salmon fillet or steak
juice of 1 lemon
1cm (½in) cube of fresh root ginger, peeled

Preheat the oven to 200°C, Gas Mark 6. Put the lemongrass on a sheet of foil and place the salmon on top. Pour the lemon juice over, then grate the ginger on top. Seal the foil package and bake in the oven for roughly 15 minutes, until cooked.

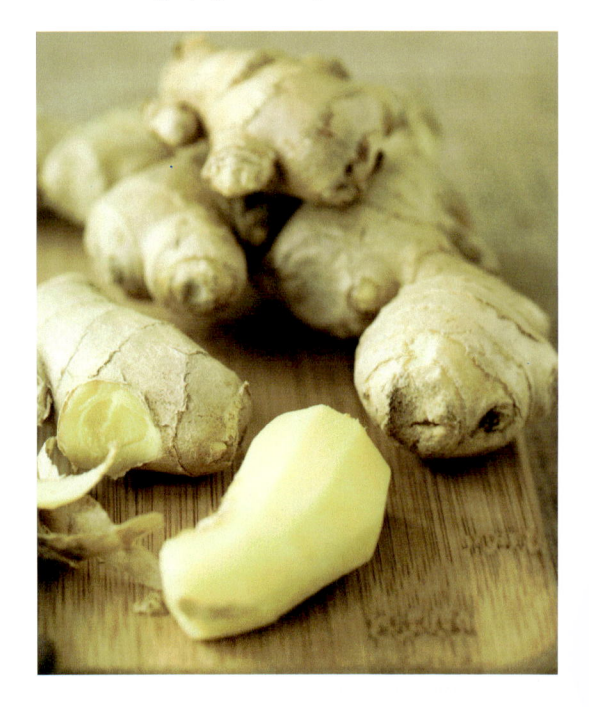

Spicy cannellini bean and tomato casserole

(*serves 2*) Serve this tasty casserole on a mound of brown rice with a large mixed green salad on the side.

Soak the cannellini beans overnight. Drain and rinse, and boil them in fresh water for 10 minutes. Drain again and set aside.

Warm the oil in a large pan and brown the onions gently. Add the garlic, cumin, coriander and chilli. Cook briefly, stirring to prevent burning, then add the beans and cover with water or vegetable stock to a depth of about 5cm (2in) – you probably need 400-500ml (14-16fl oz). Simmer for 30 minutes.

Remove the pieces of chilli unless you want a hotter dish. Add the tomatoes, red pepper, paprika, tomato purée and honey. Simmer gently for 30 minutes. The liquid should be well reduced; you may even need to add a little more (and turn the heat down) if it is vanishing too quickly. Alternatively, turn the heat up to reduce it further if you have too much; either way, you should end up with a thick sauce. Check the seasoning and serve.

Ingredients

75g (3oz) dried cannellini beans
1 tsp olive oil
2 small red onions, chopped
1 garlic clove, chopped
½ tsp ground cumin
½ tsp ground coriander
1 red chilli, halved and seeded
water or vegetable stock
2 large tomatoes, skinned and seeded
1 red pepper, seeded and chopped
½ tsp paprika
2 tsp tomato purée
2 tsp organic honey
salt and black pepper

Handling chillies

Be very careful not to touch your eyes, and wash your hands immediately after handling chillies. The seeds are the hottest part, so be thorough about removing them, and remember that chillies can vary in strength enormously, even if they come from the same pack or plant.

4 Detox recipes

Roast vegetables with sweet potato mash

(serves 1) Popularized by the GI and GL diets, sweet potatoes are a superfood with lots of the antioxidant betacarotene, and vitamins C and E to mop up free radicals.

Ingredients

1 medium sweet potato
2 tsp olive oil
250g (8oz) chopped and peeled squash, stringy centre and seeds removed
1 red onion, quartered
1 large head of fennel, sliced and broken into sections
1 red pepper, seeded and chopped
4 garlic cloves, unpeeled
1 large sprig of rosemary
juice of ½ orange
salt and black pepper

Preheat the oven to 200°C, Gas Mark 6. Bring a pan of water to the boil and drop in the whole, unpeeled sweet potato – one weighing 200g (7oz) will take about 35–45 minutes to cook.

Put the olive oil in an ovenproof dish and pop it into the oven. When it is warm, add the squash, onion, fennel and red pepper. Tuck in the garlic and scatter rosemary leaves over the top. Roast for 15 minutes, give the vegetables a good stir, and return to the oven for 10 minutes. Add salt and black pepper, give it a final stir and roast for another few minutes.

Make the mash. Drain and peel the sweet potato, then mash with a little orange juice (go easy at first and add more if necessary) and lots of black pepper. Remove the vegetables from the pan, fish out the garlic and squeeze the flesh out of the crisp skin into the sweet potato; mash it in roughly. Serve with the roasted vegetables and a crisp green salad.

Sweet potato and squash

Some varieties can become greyish if peeled before cooking, but take a chance and boil peeled sweet potato pieces for 30 minutes, until soft. Use whatever squash is available, including courgette. Butternut squash is fine, but can be quite sweet – experiment!

Masoor dhal with cauliflower

(serves 1) Curries are a fantastic detox food, as turmeric helps to avoid any problems with intermediate toxic chemicals while cumin is said to stimulate pancreatic enzymes.

Rinse and drain the lentils, checking for any small stones, and put to one side. Heat the oil in a heavy saucepan with a lid and cook the onion and garlic until they begin to brown. Add the chilli, cumin, coriander, turmeric and paprika and stir well. Stir in the lentils, then squeeze in some lemon juice. Add the cauliflower florets, 150ml (¼ pint) water or vegetable stock and the desiccated coconut.

Bring to the boil, then reduce the heat and simmer, covered, for 10 minutes. Check that there is still some liquid left, adding more if necessary, and simmer for another 5 minutes.

Add the cashews, a little salt, and most of the mint (retain some for a garnish). Simmer, uncovered, for 5 minutes until the liquid is absorbed, stirring occasionally to prevent the dhal sticking. When the lentils have formed a really thick sauce, check the seasoning and serve immediately, garnished with a few mint leaves and accompanied by a fresh cucumber salad and raw onion rings.

Ingredients

- 50g (2oz) red lentils
- 1 tsp olive oil
- 1 small onion, chopped
- 1 garlic clove, chopped
- ¼ tsp chilli powder
- ¼ tsp ground cumin
- ¼ tsp ground coriander
- ½ tsp turmeric
- ½ tsp paprika
- squeeze of lemon juice
- 1 small cauliflower (or ½ larger one), cut into medium-sized florets
- water or vegetable stock
- 10g (⅓oz) desiccated coconut
- 10g (⅓oz) cashews
- salt and black pepper
- handful of small mint leaves

4 Detox recipes

Vegetable fried rice with nori

(*serves 1*) Nori is probably more familiar to you as the seaweed frequently used to wrap sushi. It is a great source of iodine, iron, calcium and other minerals, as well as protein. If using this as an accompaniment, make half the quantity and omit the sauce, using shoyu by itself instead.

Ingredients

60g (2oz) brown basmati rice (*or* ordinary brown rice)
½ sheet of nori
1 tbsp Japanese rice vinegar
1 tbsp shoyu
½ tsp sesame oil
½ tsp grated fresh root ginger
2 tsp rapeseed oil
5 spring onions, chopped
1 carrot, chopped into 5cm (2in) fine strips
½ green pepper, seeded and chopped into fine strips
1cm (½in) cube fresh root ginger, peeled and finely chopped
1 garlic clove, finely chopped
1 tsp sesame seeds
salt and black pepper

Rinse the rice thoroughly, cover with cold water and bring to the boil. Lower the heat, cover the pan and cook gently for 20 minutes, or until it is done but retains a bit of bite. Rinse thoroughly and set aside.

Toast the nori until it changes colour and gets crisp. Crumble it into a dish. Make a sauce by whisking the rice vinegar, shoyu, sesame oil and ginger together. Put the nori and the sauce aside.

Heat 1 teaspoon rapeseed oil in a large non-stick frying pan and add the spring onions, carrot and green pepper. Fry for 5 minutes until they begin to colour, then add the ginger and garlic and cook, stirring, for 2–3 minutes.

Break up any lumps in the rice with a fork. Then add the remaining oil and the sesame seeds to the frying pan, stir thoroughly, and add the rice. Now stir continuously, heating the rice thoroughly but ensuring it does not stick, and add half the sauce. Season to taste and serve the hot rice immediately, with the toasted nori scattered over the top and the remaining sauce on the side.

Marinated vegetable kebabs

(serves 1, makes 3 skewers) These could be cooked outdoors over a barbecue while everyone else tucks into their high saturated-fat burgers and sausages. If using bamboo skewers rather than metal ones, soak them in water before you start.

Mix the marinade: put the shoyu, sesame oil, honey and garlic in a jug and stir thoroughly, then put to one side. Chop the onion into sections so that you have pieces that can be safely skewered without falling off. Seed and chop the pepper into 2.5cm (1in) chunks, and slice the courgette into rounds.

Toss these, together with the mushrooms, in the marinade. Leave for 1 hour or so.

Preheat the grill. Thread the vegetables on to the skewers, transferring any remaining marinade into a small pan (if you don't have much left, don't worry – use some plain shoyu for dipping instead).

Place the kebabs under the grill or on the barbecue and cook, being careful to turn them regularly. Warm the remaining marinade over a low heat.

Remove the kebabs from the grill or barbecue when the vegetables are beginning to brown nicely and soften, and serve with the marinade or shoyu on the side. The kebabs can be served with brown rice and a green salad made from oriental leaves.

Ingredients

1 tbsp shoyu or light soy sauce
1 tsp sesame oil
1 tsp clear honey
1 garlic clove, crushed
1 small red onion
1 yellow or red pepper
1 small courgette
6-9 button mushrooms

4 Detox recipes

Pomegranate ice

(Serves 1) Orange flower water can now be found in many health food shops, and even sometimes in supermarkets, often with the baking ingredients. It is worth getting, as it gives this dish a perfumed, Middle-Eastern touch. However, a little orange juice could be used instead.

Ingredients

½ **large pomegranate,** *or* **1 whole smaller one**
6 ice cubes
1 tbsp water
1 tsp orange flower water

Squeeze the pomegranate upside-down over a bowl to catch the juice and loosen the seeds. Still holding it upside-down in one hand, whack the skin with the back of a wooden spoon – the seeds will fall out into the bowl and any that do not can be teased out easily with a fork or the point of a sharp knife. Squeeze the skin again to extract as much juice as possible, and discard. Remove any small pieces of pith from the bowl containing the seeds and juice.

Put the ice cubes in a blender with the water and crush, using the pulse setting – alternatively, put them in a self-seal plastic bag, close it and hit them with a rolling pin. However you make your crushed ice, pile a mound of it in a serving dish (this looks wonderful in a glass bowl) and then scatter the pomegranate seeds and juice over the top; the ice will turn a delicate pale garnet colour in parts. Drizzle the orange flower water over everything and serve immediately.

Orange and date salad

(serves 1) The sharpness of the orange juice cuts through the sweetness of the dates, making this a very satisfying dessert.

Peel the orange with a knife over a bowl, removing all the pith but catching as much juice as you can. Slice it neatly. Slice the dates crosswise, quite finely. Put a few orange slices in a dish and scatter some dates over them, then add another layer of oranges. Sprinkle the remaining dates over the top, pushing them down among the oranges. Pour over the orange juice. Cover and set aside for at least 2 hours; in hot weather, store in the fridge, but bring back to room temperature before serving.

Ingredients

1 large juicy orange
4 dates

Blueberry salad

(serves 1) An antioxidant cocktail *par excellence*, and the green and purplish-black colours look very attractive in the bowl.

Pick over the blueberries and remove any bits of stalk; wash and drain them. Peel and slice the kiwi fruit and put it in a bowl with the blueberries. Wash the grapes, slice into rounds and scatter over the kiwi and blueberries. Squeeze one slice of lime into the bowl, and then cover and chill for 30 minutes. Serve, garnished with the other piece of lime.

Ingredients

75g (3oz) blueberries
1 kiwi fruit
10 black seedless grapes
2 slices of lime

4 Detox recipes

Chicken with chickpeas, olives and lemon

(serves 1) This post-detox dish uses detox foods along with organic chicken to create a perfectly satisfying meal in a pot.

Ingredients

60g (2oz) dried chickpeas
1 tsp olive oil
1 onion, chopped
½ tsp paprika
small pinch of turmeric
1 large organic chicken breast, cut into 3 or 4 chunks
200ml (7fl oz) water
juice of 1 small lemon
1 garlic clove, crushed
6-10 olives, halved
salt and black pepper
a small handful of fresh mint (optional)

Soak the chickpeas overnight, then drain and rinse. Put them in a saucepan of fresh water and boil for 10 minutes. Drain and rinse again.

Heat the olive oil in a heavy saucepan with a lid, and add the onion. When it is beginning to soften and colour, stir in the paprika and turmeric. Add the chicken and stir well to coat with the spices, then cook gently for 2 minutes.

Add the water, lemon juice, garlic and the partly-cooked chickpeas. Bring to the boil, reduce the heat and simmer gently, covered. Check after 10 minutes to make sure the liquid isn't cooking away; turn the heat down further and add more if necessary. Check again after another 15 minutes and test the chicken – it should be almost ready. Check the seasoning, add the olives and some of the mint (if using) and cook for a further 5 minutes.

When the chicken is cooked, remove it from the pan, then reduce the chickpea liquid by boiling rapidly if it's not thick enough. Once it is, spoon the chickpeas and their sauce onto a plate, arrange the chicken pieces on top and garnish with mint leaves. Serve immediately, accompanied by a green salad.

Pepper steak with two salads

(*serves 1*) When you are coming off your detox, some beef from grass-fed organically raised cows is a great source of omega-3 and iron – and it's also delicious.

Remove as much fat from the steak as possible. Grind lots of black pepper over it, pressing it into the meat. Turn it over and repeat on the other side.

Place a heavy non-stick frying pan or ridged griddle pan over a high heat, and add 1 teaspoon olive oil. While it heats up, make the salads. Put the tomatoes and onion rings in a bowl, pour over the remaining olive oil and drizzle with balsamic vinegar. Put the salad leaves into another bowl.

When the oil in the pan begins to smoke, add the steak and cook on one side. After a few minutes – how many will depend on the thickness of the steak and how you like it cooked, but it should not be more than 5 minutes – turn it over and then cook the other side.

Serve immediately the steak is done. Put the tomato salad on the plate with the meat and put the bowl with the salad leaves on the table separately. When you've eaten the steak and the tomato salad, put the leaves on your plate – the remains of the olive oil and balsamic vinegar from the tomatoes and the juices from the steak will make a delicious dressing for them.

Ingredients

1 organic sirloin steak, about 200-250g (7-8oz)
black pepper
2 tsp olive oil
2 large tomatoes, sliced
½ red onion, sliced into thin rings
balsamic vinegar
salad leaves

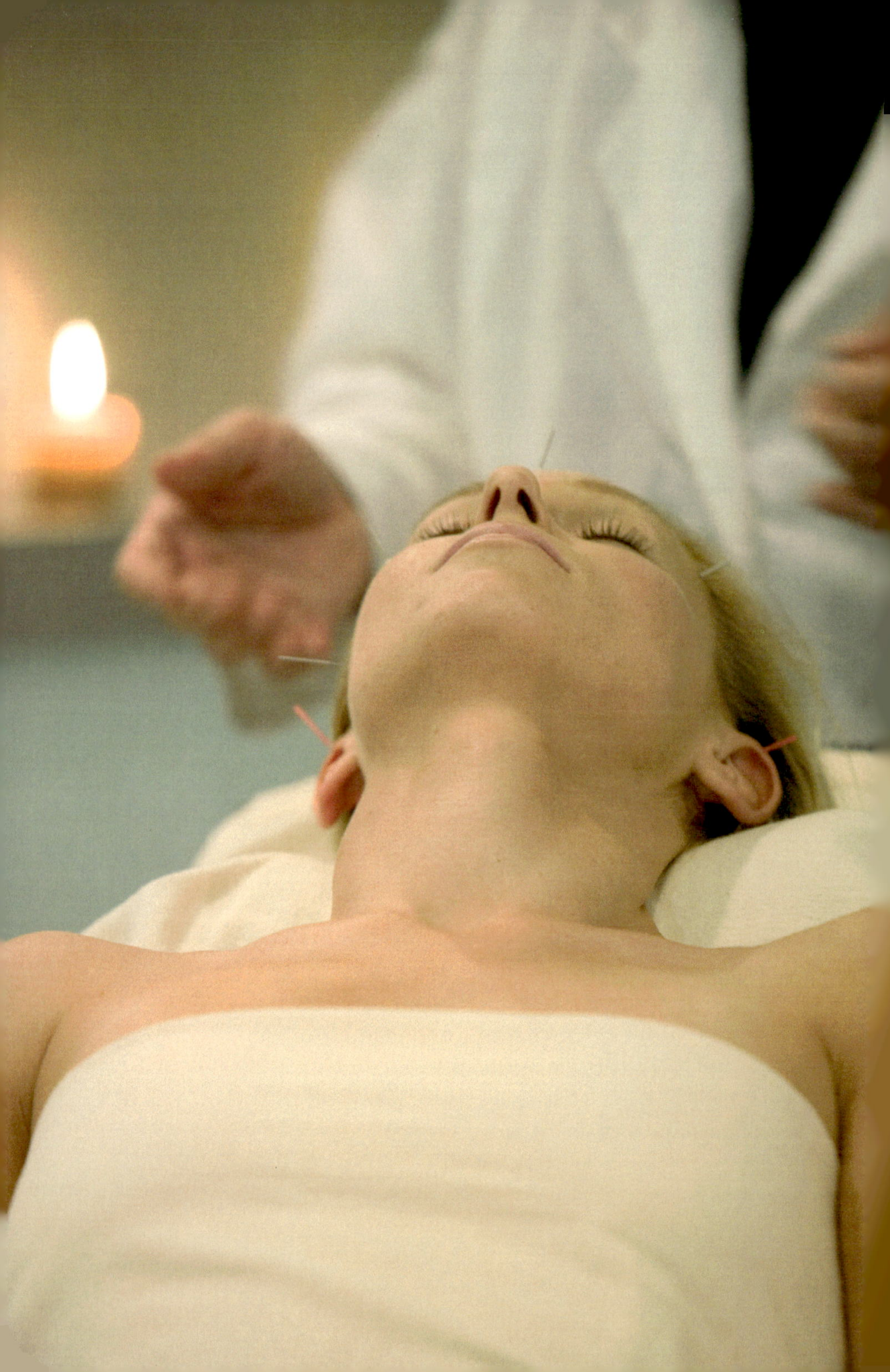

5 Detox aids

It is important to eat well when detoxing and avoid foods that challenge the system, but this is not the whole story. There are lots of other techniques that can support and intensify your detox efforts, helping you to shed more toxins and cleanse your whole system from top to toe. This chapter contains a run-down of the many treatments that you can try for yourself, in your own home, using easy-to-find products.

5 Detox aids

Supplementing your diet

Some of the treatments that are described in this chapter should be regarded as an essential part of your detox strategy, whereas others are an optional complement to it. You can either choose the treatments that address your specific symptoms, or just the ones that appeal to you.

must know

Selenium
Intensive farming has significantly decreased the levels of vital minerals in our foods over the last 30 years. It is estimated that the average person's daily intake of selenium was 60 micrograms in 1974 and is now only half of that. Selenium is an essential nutrient for helping your liver to detoxify carcinogenic chemicals. Make sure your daily supplement contains 100-200mcg.

Vitamin and mineral supplements

You should not need to take supplements if you are eating a varied diet with plenty of fresh fruits and vegetables of different colours, and lots of pulses, grains, nuts and seeds, but in practice it can be quite tricky covering all your basics.

Multivitamins

Most detox diets recommend that you take a good multivitamin and mineral supplement, which contains at least 100 per cent of the recommended daily allowance (RDA) of vitamins A to E, plus the minerals calcium, iron, zinc, magnesium, potassium and selenium.

Choose a well-known brand but read the label to watch out for any hidden ingredients, such as peanut oil, milk, gelatine, gluten, yeast or artificial flavouring and colours. Effervescent vitamins are best avoided because they can rot your teeth.

Essential fatty acids

The other supplement that you are strongly recommended to take on a detox programme is an essential fatty acid blend with omega-3 (linolenic acid) and omega-6 (linoleic acid). Essential fatty acids (EFAs) are found naturally in nuts, seeds, green leafy vegetables, whole grains and oily fish but it is estimated that eight out of ten people do not get enough from their diet. EFAs are essential for the production of prostaglandins that balance metabolic reactions, and imbalances can cause a range of symptoms such as skin rashes, frequent thirst, dry hair and skin, low sex drive and a lowered immunity to infections. Take 500–1000mg of evening primrose oil, 1–4g of a fish oil supplement or a dessertspoon of flaxseed oil. Udo's oil, which is available from health food shops and complementary chemists, is a good mix.

Herbal supplements

Made from the roots, stems, leaves, flowers, sap, bark, fruit and seeds of different plants, herbal supplements can be powerful detox helpers, stimulating liver and kidney function and protecting your organs and tissues from released toxins. Herbalists prefer to use tinctures made by soaking the herbs in an alcohol base, but you may find it more convenient to take tablets or capsules, made from dried or powdered extracts of the active component of the herb. You can also drink teas prepared from dried herbs, although the dosage will not be exact in this instance.

When buying herbs, do look out for 'standardized' extracts which tell you how much of the active ingredient is present in each dose. Many cheap, non-standardized preparations contain very little.

It's not advisable to take more than one herb at a time except under the supervision of a qualified herbalist, as there might be interactions (although

must know

Taking supplements
Supplements should normally be taken after a meal and washed down with water. Don't take them with tea or coffee, as this could interfere with their absorption. If it's a one-a-day supplement, take it after the evening meal rather than breakfast, so it can do its work during the night when a lot of repair processes take place in the body.

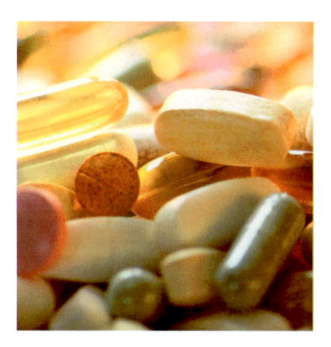

Check the sell-by dates when buying supplements. The older they are, the lower the potency.

5 Detox aids

you can drink herbal teas quite safely). Don't take herbs at all, without discussing it first with your doctor or specialist, if you are on any prescribed medication or have a chronic illness or health condition. For information on finding a herbalist or buying herbs by mail order, see page 131. Below is a selection of the best detox herbal supplements, their uses and the dose you should take.

Echinacea

If you are prone to colds or the flu virus, try this immune system booster as part of your detox plan. Studies have shown that people taking echinacea get half as many infections as those who don't, and the ones they get tend to be less severe. It promotes

Echinacea is thought to work by stimulating the white blood cells that mop up bacteria and viruses.

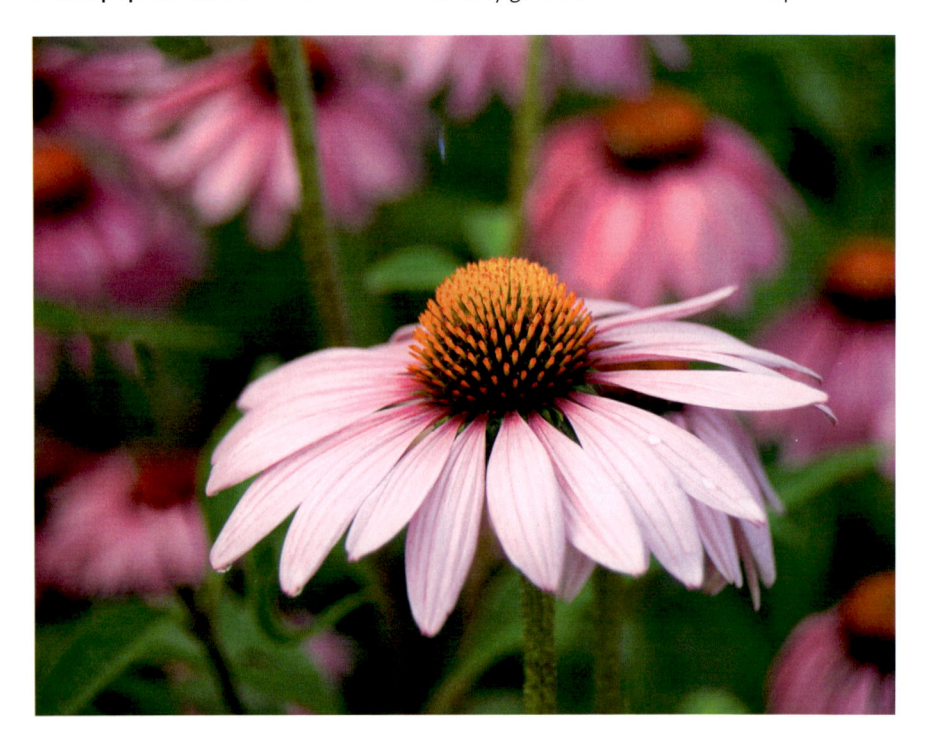

sweating and can help with chronic fatigue syndrome following a viral infection. Take a 500mg tablet or 20 drops of tincture a day during a detox to help with cleansing. If you do get a cold or flu, take 300mg three times a day to help fight it off.

Milk thistle

The most famous detox herb, and rightly so. More than 300 studies have now shown that its active ingredient, silymarin, can protect liver cells from the poisonous effects of alcohol and other toxic chemicals. It inhibits free radical formation and boosts glutathione levels in the liver by over 33 per cent. It prevents poisons from penetrating the liver cells and also stimulates them to regenerate after cell damage. If you are not taking any other detox herbs to treat specific symptoms, choose this popular detox aid. Start with a dose of 100mg taken three times a day, standardized to at least 70 per cent silymarin, or take 20 drops of milk thistle tincture in water.

Artichoke extract

Globe artichoke is related to milk thistle. A number of studies have shown that artichoke leaf extracts can reduce the effects of excess alcohol, lower cholesterol, increase bile secretion and improve digestive symptoms such as bloating and flatulence. In a study of 550 people taking artichoke extracts for 66 weeks, abdominal pain was reduced by 76 per cent, constipation by 71 per cent and bloating by 66 per cent. If you experience a lot of digestive system problems, try taking standardized 320mg capsules one to three times a day with food.

---

must know

Ancient detox aids
Native Americans, such as the Sioux, have long used echinacea to counteract the toxins from rattlesnake bites and scorpion stings. Back in the fifteenth century, European mushroom gatherers knew that milk thistle could help you survive if you ate a bad mushroom. The sixteenth-century herbalist John Gerard advised stepchildren to have lemons handy in case they were poisoned by their stepmothers.

5 Detox aids

Buchu
The leaves of this aromatic herb are diuretic and stimulate kidney cells to flush toxins from your body more quickly. Buchu has antibacterial properties that combat urinary tract infections and it helps to prevent kidney stones. You can buy buchu leaves with which to make a tea from most good health food shops, or buy ready-made teabags. You can also buy buchu tincture. Try this if you don't urinate very often or you have a history of urinary tract infections, to make sure that your kidneys function effectively during a detox.

Dandelion
If you have a sluggish digestion and are prone to constipation, this should be your detox aid of choice. It stimulates the liver to increase the flow of bile and has a gentle laxative action. It is also good for addressing hormone imbalances that are caused by oestrogen dominance, with symptoms such as cyclical breast pain in women. Drink three cups of dandelion tea or coffee a day or buy standardized 500mg extracts or tincture.

Ashwaganda
This is the supplement for you if you have a high-stress lifestyle. Studies suggest that it prevents the depletion of vitamin C and cortisol during periods of stress, reduces anxiety and promotes refreshing sleep. It boosts immunity and energy levels and can act as an aphrodisiac, counteracting impotence in men. Take two 250mg capsules a day or mix dried root powder with some boiling water and honey. Try the stress-reducing techniques in Chapter 8 as well.

---

must know

Laxatives
Avoid buying strong laxatives, such as senna or dock, or mixtures containing them, if you suffer from constipation. The results may be rapid but the resultant speed of bowel movements can cause you to lose important nutrients and it is possible to become so dependent on laxatives that you are unable to have a normal bowel movement without them. Increase your fibre intake as a first course of action, then try dandelion tea; if this doesn't work, take aloe vera juice. Experiment until you find the combination that helps you pass the stools test on page 23.

Schisandra

If you have to take prescription drugs, work with toxic chemicals or have a problem with alcohol abuse, this can protect the liver and speed toxin removal from the body. The berries are the detoxification agent and can be taken as a tea or in extracts of 300mg. It might be worth taking schisandra preventively before painting your house or adding fertilizer to the garden, to raise your resistance to the toxins you'll be exposed to. (See Chapter 8 for alternatives to common household products.)

Panax ginseng

For those with a history of smoking, heavy drinking or taking street, OTC or prescription drugs, ginseng can be used to protect the body from cancers and reduce the damage caused by long-term exposure to the toxins in these substances. Don't take it if you have high blood pressure. You are advised to take ginseng for two weeks on, two weeks off. Choose a standardized product with no less than 5 per cent ginsenosides and start with around 600mg a day. Alternatively, boil 1 teaspoon of dried root for 10-20 minutes to make a tea, or take 20 drops root tincture.

Aloe vera

Fresh aloe vera juice, found in good health food shops, is a powerful tool for rectifying intestinal problems like bloating, flatulence, constipation and irritable bowel syndrome. Start with a small (50ml) daily dose or follow the guidelines on the product. Some people find the laxative effect of pure juice too powerful. You can also buy aloe vera tablets; one brand is sold under the label 'Colon Cleanse'.

> **must know**
>
> **Aloe vera gel**
> This can be helpful for treating skin conditions, e.g. eczema, psoriasis and sunburn, as it soothes and stimulates tissue regeneration in the area. In one study of 60 adults with psoriasis, those using aloe vera gel found that 80 per cent of rashes healed while only eight per cent noticed an improvement in the placebo group. Try it if you have reactive skin, but stop if it feels as though it is irritating it.

5 Detox aids

Exercising during a detox

Moderate-intensity exercise will boost your detox programme on different levels. You can choose a mixture of aerobic exercise, a heart/lung workout that leaves you out of breath and sweating, and anaerobic exercise, designed to build muscle strength.

must know

Walking
Dawdling along the high street window-shopping and daydreaming does not count as exercise. If you want walking to be one of your daily detox exercises, you need to walk briskly, rolling from the heel through the foot and pushing off with the toes. Wear flat shoes with flexible soles that allow you to do this.

Opposite: Joining an exercise class can help provide motivation through group support.

Reasons to exercise

Here are the top 10 reasons to exercise during your detox. They are listed in no particular order – we all have different weak areas.

1 Most people only breathe from the top third of their lungs, meaning that stale air and waste carbon dioxide stagnate lower down. Exercise that stimulates you to breathe deeply, using the whole of your lung capacity, will clear out the waste gases and let more oxygen cross the barrier into your bloodstream. If you don't feel out of breath during an aerobic exercise session, you're not working hard enough.

2 Aerobic exercise makes your heart beat faster, pumping oxygenated blood round your system and through your liver and kidneys. Your cells are thus cleansed of waste materials and supplied with nutrients more efficiently.

3 Both aerobic and anaerobic exercises get your lymphatic system moving, taking white blood cells to sites where they are needed and filtering out toxins from the tissues, thus helping to shift cellulite.

4 Exercise burns fat, releasing stored toxins into the bloodstream where they can be excreted through the liver, kidneys, lungs or skin.

5 Exercise that increases the amount you sweat will help you to release toxins through the skin,

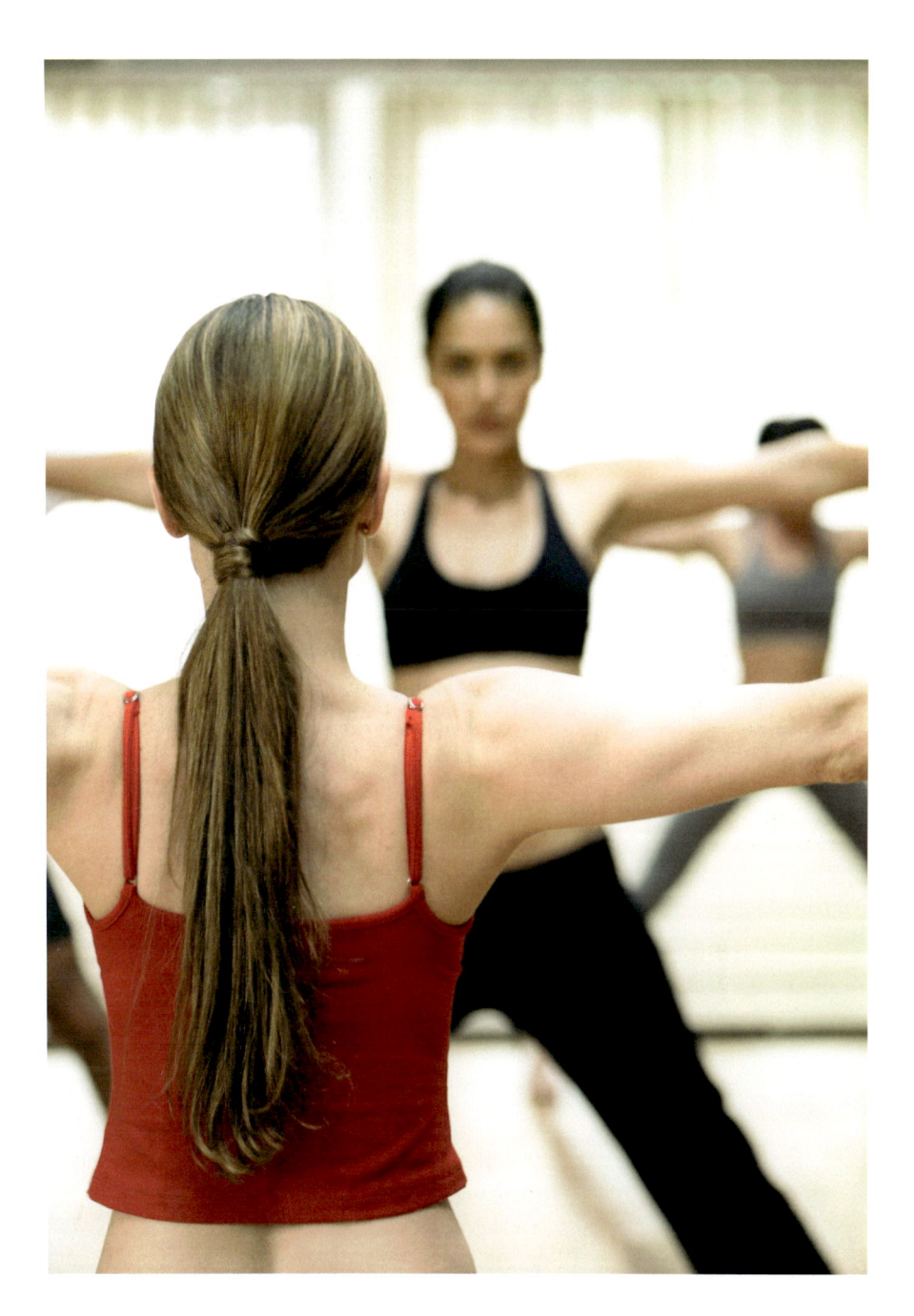

5 Detox aids

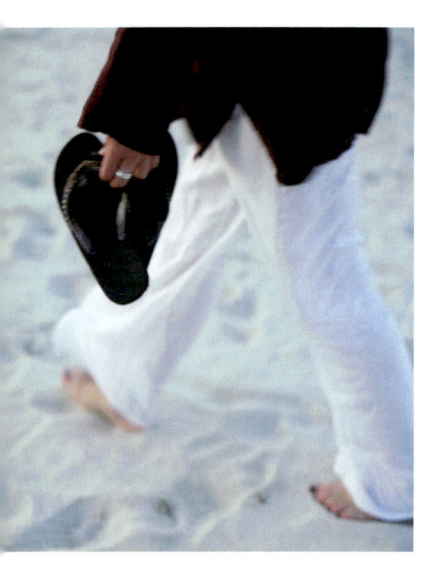

Walking barefoot on sand is a great workout for leg muscles.

including heavy metals, pesticides and pollutants.

6 Exercise stimulates the immune system to produce more disease-fighting cells. In a study of 150 people, those who walked on a regular basis contracted about half the number of colds as those who didn't.

7 Exercise can stimulate bowel movements as the movement of the outer, voluntary muscles provokes contraction of the inner, involuntary ones.

8 Exercise is a powerful mood enhancer and de-stresser, causing the brain to release feel-good chemicals, burning off stress hormones, lowering blood pressure and promoting restful sleep.

9 From our mid-30s onwards, hormonal changes cause us to lose muscle mass and store more fat, unless we combat this process with exercise. When you lose muscle, you burn fewer calories and put on weight even if you are eating the same amount of food you always did. More weight equals more toxins. By doing regular strength-training exercise, you can keep the muscles you had and even replace lost muscle.

10 Exercise makes you look better. Your muscles will be more toned, your belly flattened and skin tone improved. If no other reason from this list motivates you, then exercise for the sake of vanity!

What kind of exercise?

The best exercise for you is the one that you enjoy the most and which fits in best with your lifestyle.

• Aerobic exercises include tennis, football and other ball sports; running and fast walking; skipping rope, trampolining, dance classes, swimming, cycling, skiing, skating and aerobic exercise classes (such as step or spinning).

- Anaerobic exercises include weight training in a gym, either on the equipment or with free weights; stretching; all kinds of yoga, and Pilates. If you do an aerobic session one day, then do an anaerobic one the next. As little as 20 minutes a day will make a difference, although up to an hour is even better.

Do not ever launch into an extreme exercise programme when you are detoxing, as this will direct the blood to your muscles rather than your detoxification organs and could release more toxins than your body is able to cope with, making you feel quite unwell.

Yoga promotes flexibility, which becomes increasingly important as we age. It is worth trying if you still want to be able to put your own socks on at sixty.

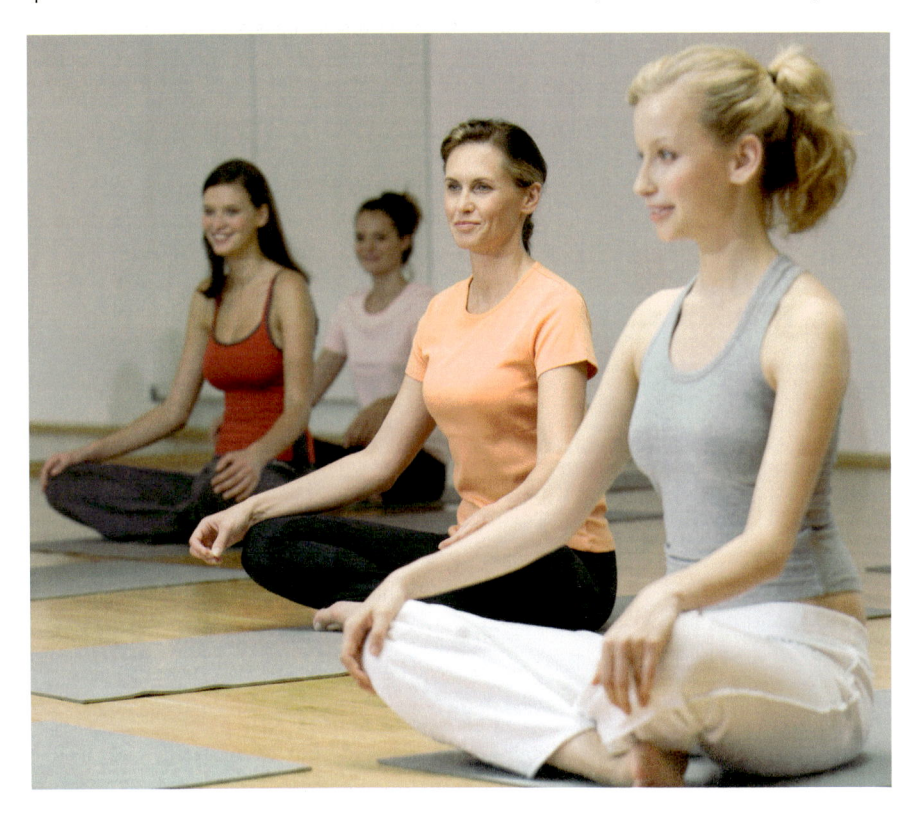

5 Detox aids

Your daily bathing routine

Dry skin brushing should be a part of every detox programme. It feels fantastic and is a great way of sloughing off dead skin cells and toxins excreted in sweat, as well as stimulating the lymphatic system and the blood circulation. Buy a soft, natural-bristle skin brush and use it once a day before you shower or bathe.

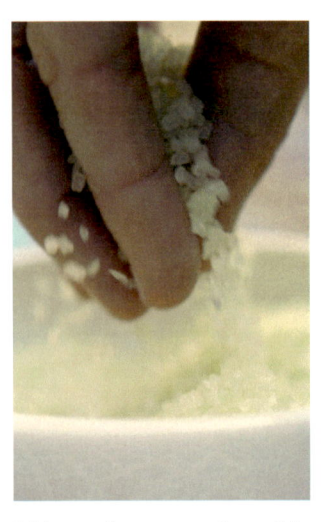

Add around a quarter of a cupful of bath salts to your bath.

Dry skin brushing

It is important when dry skin brushing to avoid any areas with broken skin as you work. The whole routine should take you around five minutes.

1 First, undress completely. Sitting on the edge of the bath, start brushing the sole of the left foot, then the left leg from the foot to the knee, with long, firm strokes.

2 When you have finished the lower leg, stand up and brush from the knee to the top of the thigh and over the buttocks. Repeat with the right leg.

3 Next brush your left arm from the palm of the hand up to the wrist, and then up to the shoulder. Repeat with the right arm.

4 Brush your stomach, using gentle clockwise movements, then brush your back from the bottom up, and then the top down.

5 Don't brush your face – instead, rub it with a dry flannel.

Showering or bathing

When you have finished brushing, have your shower or bath, using salts, seaweed or oils, as you wish. Make the water as hot as you can take it to create perspiration, then finish with a cool shower or rinse to increase the circulation and invigorate the lymphatic system. Just one minute under a cool shower or splashing yourself with cold water will make a big difference, so don't be a wimp about it.

Bath salts

Mineral salts encourage perspiration when they are added to the bath or used as an exfoliant scrub. Choose from Epsom salts, Dead Sea salts, Celtic Sea salts, or any other kind of marine salt you can find – but not ordinary table salt.

Rub salts over your skin, using gentle, circular movements and then shower off thoroughly.

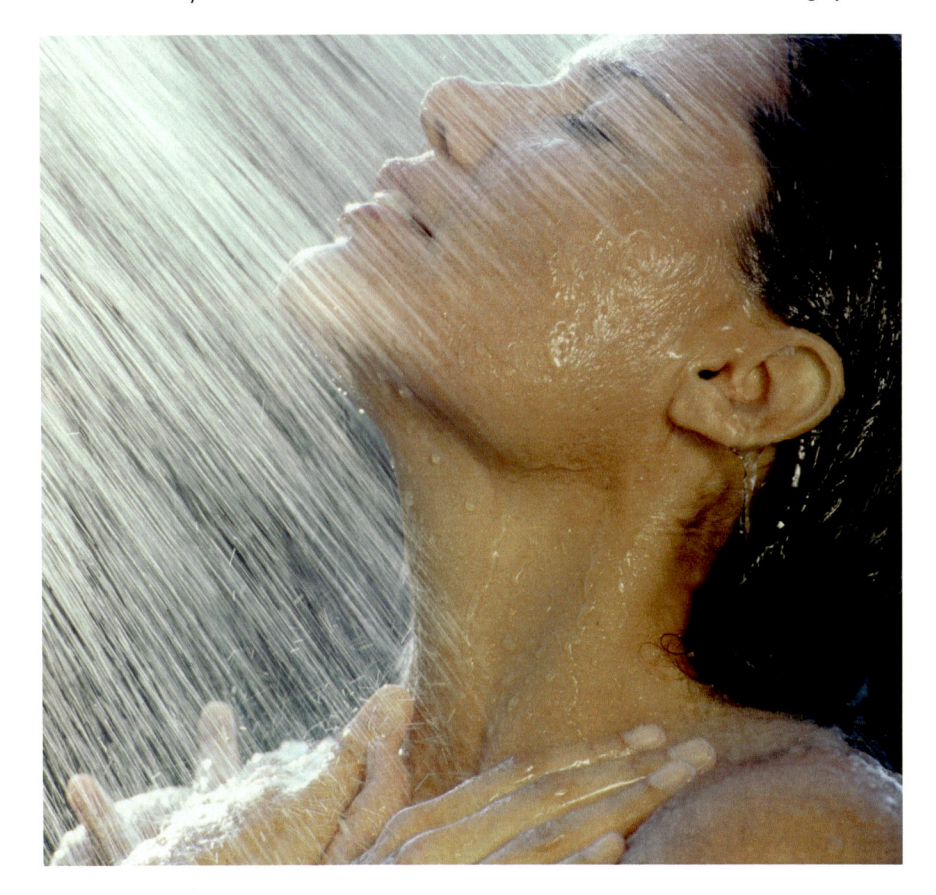

5 Detox aids

> **must know**
>
> **Detoxing oils**
> • To encourage the body to detox: juniper, lavender, geranium and rosemary.
> • To relieve headaches: rosemary, peppermint and lavender.
> • To help relieve stress: geranium, sandalwood, rose or ylang-ylang.
> • To stimulate the circulation: cypress, juniper, thyme or rose.
> • For insomnia: clary-sage, camphor, Roman chamomile, lavender, rose, sandalwood or ylang-ylang might help when added to a pre-bedtime bath.

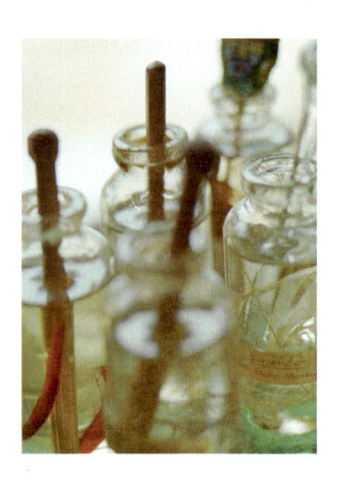

Dissolve them in the bath water and then lie back and relax in the bath for at least five minutes before using a loofah or a brush to scrub away all the perspiration the salts have drawn out. Alternatively, make a salt scrub by mixing your salt with olive oil and your choice of aromatherapy oil.

Seaweed baths

Seaweed contains large quantities of minerals, including calcium, phosphorus, magnesium, iron, iodine and sodium. It also contains acids that can draw toxins through the pores of the skin. Therapeutic seaweed is available either in dried or powdered form from chemists. Steep it in the bathwater in a muslin bag or an infusion ball. Alternatively, you can also buy a seaweed gel that you apply all over your body before a bath. It's much cheaper than the seaweed wraps you are offered in fancy spas but often just as effective.

Aromatherapy oils

Essential oils from aromatic plants have many therapeutic properties and some of them are ideal for intensifying a detox programme and/or dealing with detox side effects such as headaches and fatigue. There are several ways to use oils – in an aromatherapy burner, in a compress, for a massage, or to inhale in steam from a bowl of hot water – but one of the easiest is to add 5–10 drops of essential oil to a warm bath. Don't apply oils neat to the skin; always mix them with a carrier oil such as sweet almond, sunflower or apricot kernel oil (about 10 drops essential oil to 2 tablespoons carrier oil). To find an aromatherapist, see the box on page 131.

Other detox aids

You now have all the elements you need for a good basic detox programme, but there are several more detox helpers that can speed the process along, including flower essences, foot patches and special detox kits that are on sale in many pharmacies.

Flower essences

Flower remedies are the concentrated essence of particular flowers dissolved in an alcohol base. They are designed to help with specific mental states, especially negative emotions, and the theory is that if you heal the mind, the body will follow. Deciding which flower remedy to take depends on analysing your own mental state or getting a therapist who specializes in flower essences to do it for you.

You take flower essences by dotting them on to your pulse points 4–6 times a day, dotting them on your tongue, or by drinking a few drops in a glass of water. The amount of alcohol you will ingest this way is tiny but if you want to be completely alcohol free during your detox, then stick with the pulse method. For information and advice on flower remedies and which to use, see below.

> **must know**
>
> **Flower remedies**
> • For more information and advice on all flower remedies, log on to: http://flowervr.com/
> • To buy the flower remedies by mail order, you can call Flower Essence Repertoire (01428 741672) or ring Nelson's Pharmacy (020 7495 2404).

Types of essence
• Bush Flower Essences Purifying Essence is specifically designed for detoxing, both physically and emotionally. It should help you to let go of emotional baggage and leave you feeling relieved and cleansed. Its exotic-sounding ingredients are Bush Iris, Bottlebrush, Dagger Hakea, Dog Rose and Wild Potato Bush.

5 Detox aids

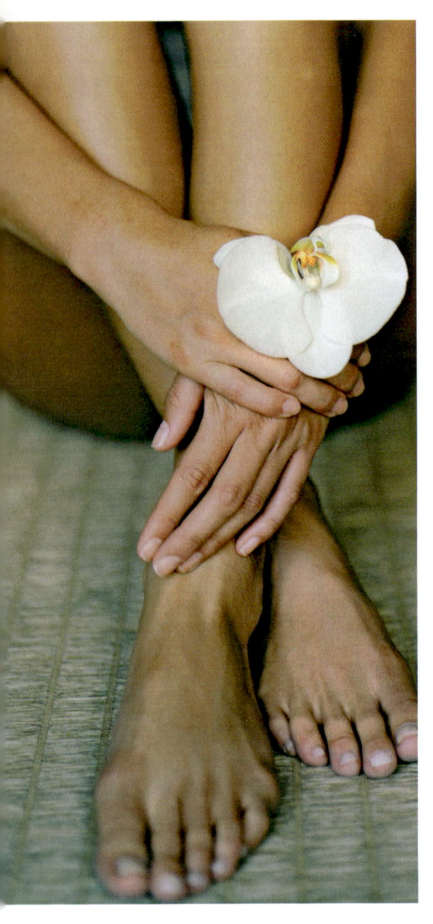

- Bush Flowers Mountain Devil is also good for detoxification and deep cleansing of the system, particularly if you are feeling angry and irritable.
- Bach Flowers Rescue Remedy is an excellent handbag standby to relieve headaches and problems with concentration or grogginess.
- Bach Flowers Crab Apple is also a cleansing remedy for those who feel unclean or polluted, physically or emotionally.
- Yarrow flower essence is said to detoxify and strengthen the body.

Foot patches

According to Chinese medicine, the body has over 360 acupuncture points with more than 60 on the soles of the feet. Foot patches containing a blend of mineral and clay powders draw out toxins through the soles of the feet, taking the pressure off your liver, kidneys and other detox organs. They help release blockages in the lymphatic system, clear nerve pathways and accelerate toxin release in the blood.

Before you go to sleep at night, tape a white detox pad to the soles of your feet. You may be aware of a slight burning, throbbing sensation, but it's not uncomfortable. When you wake up in the morning, the pads will be brown and sticky with all the toxins they have drawn out of you as you slept.

Claims made for the foot patches include improving blood circulation, increasing metabolism, relieving joint pain, enhancing the quality of sleep, relieving stress and tension, and removing toxins. Whether you believe this or not, you'll be amazed at the gunk that appears on your foot patches and relieved to have the toxins outside your body rather than inside.

The feet are an important area for toxin release. Regular foot baths can help the process.

Detox kits

You may have seen these for sale in chemists and mail order magazines. They often contain different supplements for you to take during the first half and second half of your detox, so there is a 'cleansing' and then a 'restoring' phase. Typically, the cleansing supplements will contain milk thistle, dandelion, burdock root, kelp powder and psyllium, among other substances. The restoration supplements will include lactobacillus or other probiotics, beetroot juice, and more milk thistle. There is nothing wrong with using a detox kit if you are in good health and not taking any other medications, but you may find the levels of active ingredients you consume are not as high as if you bought the individual herbs.

What should you take?

The essential detox rules are as follows:
- Only eat detox foods.
- Drink 2 litres (3½ pints) of water a day and as many herb teas as you like.
- Take a good multivitamin and mineral supplement, plus an essential fatty acid supplement.
- Take milk thistle or another herb to suit your symptoms.
- Exercise for at least 20 minutes a day.
- Dry brush your skin once a day before bathing.
- As for the foot patches, aromatherapy oils and flower essences, it's entirely up to you. If you can afford it, try them all and see what you think works.
- In the next chapter there are a number of spa treatments that are offered specifically to help detox efforts – once again, the choice is yours.

want to know more?

- For mail order herbs, call Neals' Yard Remedies (0845 2623145), Victoria Health (0800 413596), The Nutri Centre (0800 587 2290) or Napiers (0131 343 6683).
- To buy aromatherapy oils by mail order, call Neal's Yard Remedies (0845 2623145) or log on: www.nealsyardremedies.com

weblinks

- To find a herbalist, contact the National Institute of Medical Herbalists on 01392 426022, or log on to: www.nimh.org.uk
- To find a local aromatherapist, contact the Aromatherapy Consortium (0870 7743477) or log on to: www.aromatherapy-regulation.org.uk
- To order foot patches, call Ph99 Group (0800 849 6763) or look at: www.detoku.com

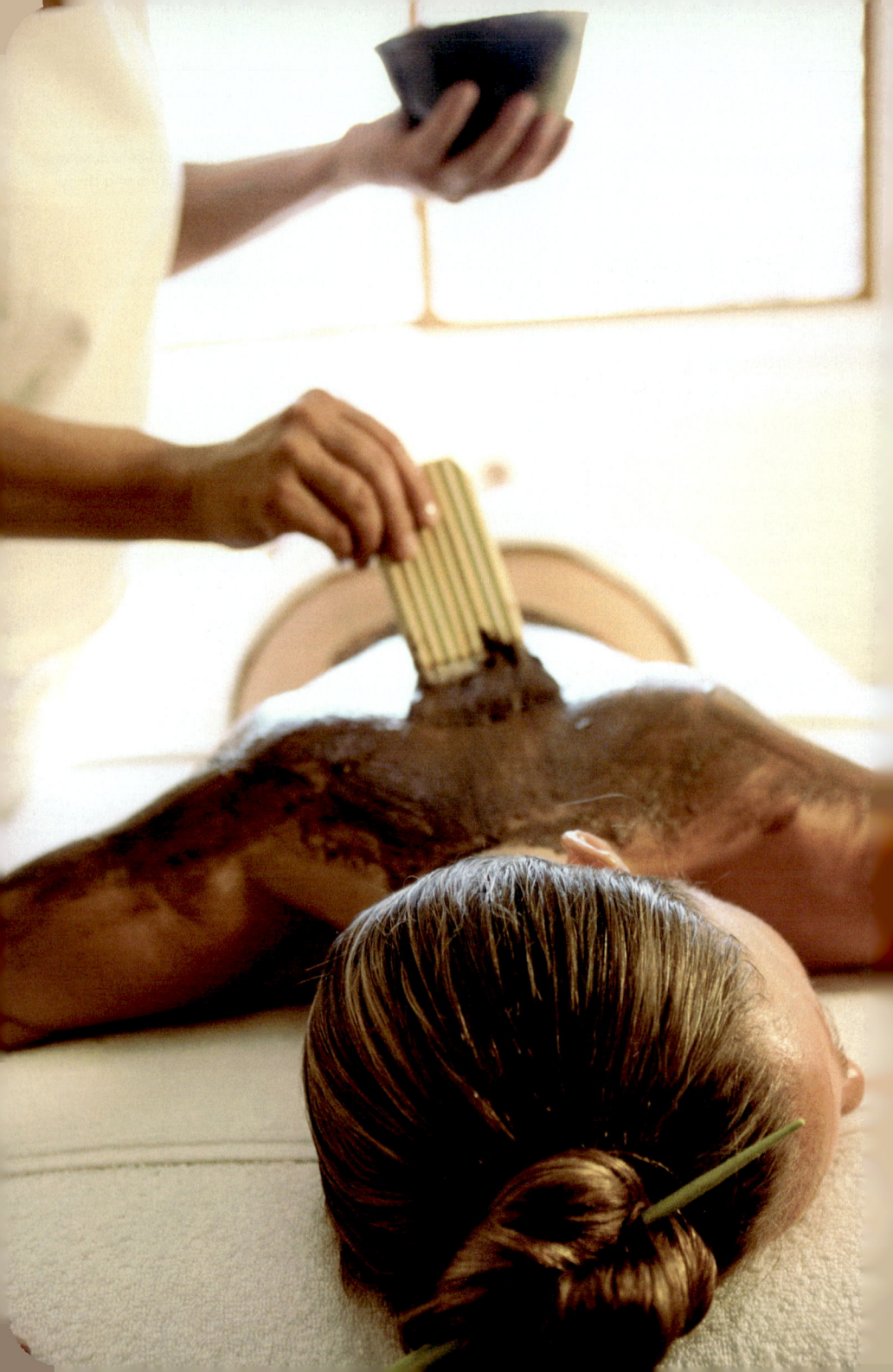

6 Holistic detox therapies

None of the therapies described in this chapter are essential on a detox programme but they would probably all help you to shed more of your toxin load. Some are extremely enjoyable, whereas others are decidedly not. The facts are here and it's up to you to decide. A really pleasant way to detox is to travel to one of the exotic spa locations that now offer a range of treatments in beautiful sunny surroundings. Read up on the therapies here first and you will know what you are letting yourself in for.

6 Holistic detox therapies

Choosing a therapy

Most of the therapies in this chapter should only be carried out by a trained professional. Don't try them by yourself at home and avoid them if you have any kind of medical condition, or if you are pregnant, unless you are specifically referred by your doctor.

> **must know**
>
> **Spa holidays**
> At the following website, www.andalucia.com/health/alternative-health, you will find descriptions of over 50 different alternative therapies by health journalist Dee McMath, who has personally tried most of them. If you've ever wondered what Okkaido or Harmonic Resonance Therapy involve, here's your chance to find out.

Chelation

Some alternative practitioners recommend this process for those people who have a build-up of heavy metals in their blood and tissues. Chelation is only performed in specialist clinics, where an intravenous drip is used to deliver 'chelating agents' which bind heavy metals, such as nickel, lead, mercury, cadmium and arsenic, and then pull them out through the stools, sweat and urine.

Chelating agents were first used during World War I to counteract the arsenic-based poison gas used in the trenches. They have also been used to treat people who are suffering from exposure to lead-based paints, or who have been contaminated with radioactivity. A clinical trial is taking place to examine the effectiveness of chelation in the treatment of atherosclerosis (narrowing of the arteries due to the build-up of cholesterol and other substances), but this will not report until 2008.

Should you try chelation?
Chelation is quite an extreme treatment and should be approached only with great care. Check the qualifications of any clinic or practitioner offering it. You will not currently be referred for chelation on

the NHS in the UK, but the British Heart Foundation is keeping an open mind about its possible benefits in the treatment of heart disease.

If you go to a clinic for chelation therapy to treat heavy metal toxicity, you will need between 10 and 40 sessions, depending on the level of toxins they detect in your initial tests. An intravenous drip will be put in your arm, containing vitamins, minerals and a chelating agent, and you will be told to lie back. Magnesium-based drips take between one and four hours but new calcium drips take just 15 minutes per session. You may feel tired and/or dizzy afterwards as your blood pressure may drop, so arrange for someone to pick you up from the clinic rather than trying to drive yourself home. Of course, this therapy will work out to be quite expensive, given the length of time it takes, the number of sessions, and the experienced medical supervision you will need to receive.

Colonic irrigation

In use since ancient Egyptian times, colonic irrigation is an effective method of getting rid of waste from a clogged-up colon by washing it out with water. Here's what happens at a session.

A trained therapist will go over your medical history first and ask you to change into a gown. You then lie on your side with your knees up and a speculum connected to sterile rubber tubing is inserted into your rectum. You lie on your back with your knees bent and the water is turned on. You are asked to hold it in for as long as it feels comfortable, then the therapist releases the pressure, allowing the water and accumulated waste to flow away.

must know

Finding a therapist
It should be relatively easy to find a colonic irrigation therapist, as most complementary health clinics will offer this service. To be registered to practise in the UK, a therapist must have trained in anatomy and physiology plus a body-based therapy, and they must also have taken a course at an approved hydrotherapy training school. Check before you get on the treatment table!

6 Holistic detox therapies

must know

Coffee enemas
Certain spas offer enema treatments, or you can buy your own enema kit in pharmacies or over the internet, but the coffee enema, generally used for detox purposes, is quite a harsh one. Coffee grounds irritate the muscles of the colon, encouraging it to contract and squeeze out its contents. The caffeine is quickly absorbed through the veins of the rectum and taken in the blood up to the liver where, it is claimed, it dilates the bile ducts, stimulating toxins to be passed into the intestine and thus expelled.

The therapist will massage your lower abdomen to help with the elimination process. The flushing is repeated until the water runs clear, or until the therapist feels that you have had enough. At the first session, you might release waste equivalent to 20-30 bowel movements, as the entire 2-metre (6-ft) length of the colon is cleansed.

From the waste evacuated, the therapist should be able to advise you on modifications to your diet which will improve your digestion. They will say, for example, if you need to eat more fibre or less fat or sugar. The first session will usually last for 30-45 minutes and you may be advised to return at a later date for more treatments. After a session, you should take probiotic supplements to replace intestinal bacteria that have been washed away.

What are the effects?
Most people feel distinctly healthier after colonic irrigation, and you may find that your weight has dropped by several pounds without those clogged-up waste materials. Your digestive system will function more effectively, as will the liver and kidneys. If you were prone to headaches, you might find they clear up now, and many people claim to sleep better. However, the effects might not be particularly long-lasting.

Detoxing holidays

If you want to combine detoxing with a holiday, you can book into a spa resort that offers a complete detox package in idyllic surroundings. You might fast during the week, taking in only detox cocktails (psyllium husk and clay, for example), herbal laxatives and one daily bowl of vegetable broth. You will also be taught how to administer your own daily coffee enema and may even be encouraged to sift through the evacuated waste material to see what comes out. Guests at such detox resorts have described finding tapeworms, liver flukes, huge chunks of undigested meat, yellow fatty deposits and string-like shreds of various hues.

After a week of fasting, raw fruits and vegetables may be consumed for the next few days. Everyone loses weight and emerges with clear, glowing skin and improved digestion, but whether they keep the weight off will depend on the eating habits they maintain on their return from holiday. Certainly, sifting through your own waste materials can help to put you off eating unhealthily, but it is not to everyone's taste.

Traditional Chinese Medicine

Chinese therapists see good health as a harmonious balance in the body between the forces of *yin* and *yang*, with energy known as *chi* flowing freely along meridians. If *chi* becomes blocked or imbalanced, illness can result. In Chinese medicine, detoxification involves removing 'devil toxins', which include heat, cold, parasites, damp, fire and food toxins.

At an initial consultation, the therapist will look at your general appearance, examine your tongue, ask questions about your lifestyle and medical history, and take your pulses from three positions on each wrist. Depending on the diagnosis, they may decide to treat you with acupuncture, in which case thin needles are inserted at the acupoints along the meridians to free blockages and stimulate the flow

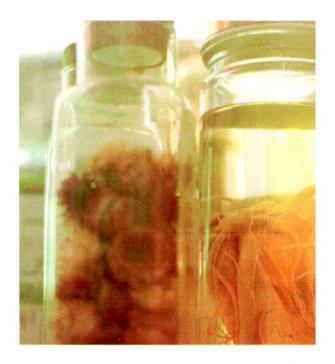

Chinese herbs are prescribed to rebalance the elements in the body.

must know

Harsh regimes
Most complementary therapists would probably advise against 'short, sharp shock' treatments, opting for gradual dietary changes and recommending colonic irrigation only if there is a large build-up of waste in the colon. An enema only cleanses the lower 20-30cm of the bowel, while colonics will cleanse the entire 2 metres (6 ft) and use a lot more water, but you are certainly not advised to try colonics at home as you could seriously injure delicate tissues.

6 Holistic detox therapies

> **must know**
>
> **Auriculotherapy**
> In this form of Chinese acupuncture, little pins are inserted at the acupoints in the ear. It is a powerful method of treating addictions of all kinds, from drugs to alcohol to smoking. When a craving comes on, you twiddle the pin or pins to stimulate the appropriate acupoint, which reactivates the treatment and helps to stop you backsliding.

of *chi*. You might be offered herbal detoxification formulas designed to boost the metabolism to burn fats and clean up the digestive system. These remedies could be herbs with which you brew teas, or pills, powders or pastes. Some therapists use a combination of acupuncture and herbs, as required. There will usually be follow-up sessions to chart progress and adjust the treatments according to the way in which the body is responding.

What can it treat?

Traditional Chinese Medicine (TCM) is especially recommended for treating digestive disorders, such as irritable bowel syndrome; chronic skin conditions like eczema; fatigue and depression; hormonal imbalances such as PMS; endometriosis and poor sperm count, and infertility (both male and female). It can produce results with chronic conditions that Western methods fail to help.

Self-diagnosis and treatment of medical conditions are not recommended, but at some TCM centres you can describe your symptoms to the practitioner behind the counter and receive an appropriate remedy on the spot. TCM can be very successful for treating people undergoing withdrawal from drug and alcohol addictions. Alcohol creates liver and gall bladder imbalances, which brings about a combination of excessive dampness and heat. Many drugs are processed through the liver, making it heated and congested so the liver blood becomes weak and deficient. TCM formulas focus on clearing and nourishing the liver and gall bladder, while at the same time treating the heart, to help calm the mind and nervous system.

Ayurvedic detoxification

Ayurveda is an ancient Indian system of healthcare and, like Chinese medicine, it is based on the idea of balance within the body. There are three primary *doshas* – *kapha*, *pitta* and *vata* – of which we all have different degrees in our bodies and personalities, and treating symptoms of unwellness will involve balancing the *doshas*.

Ayurveda is a complete holistic system which should only be followed under the supervision of a qualified practitioner. The main method of detoxification, which is called *Panchakarma*, works on several levels. First, your diet is cleared out and

A skilled therapist can feel any blockages in your system and diagnose problems by touching.

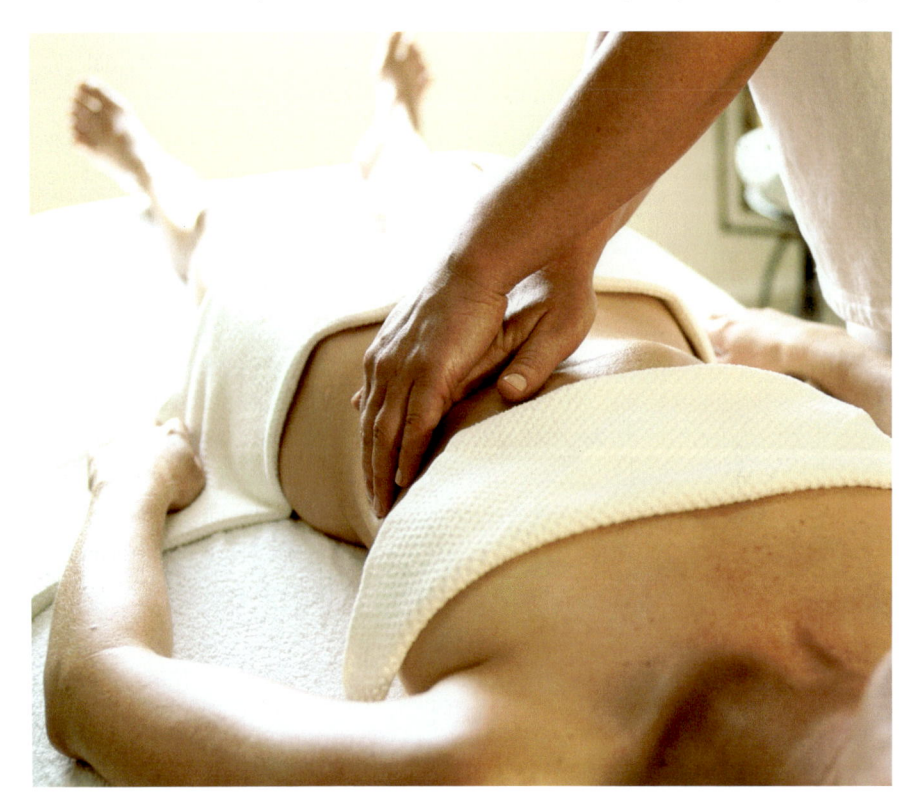

6 Holistic detox therapies

> **must know**
>
> **The doshas**
> Our constitution is determined by the state of our parents' *doshas* at the moment we are conceived. We all have a balance of the three:
> • *Vata* is the driving force, relating to energy and the nervous system.
> • *Pitta* is fire, relating to metabolism, digestion, enzymes and bile.
> • *Kapha* is related to water in the mucous membranes, phlegm, fat and lymphatic system.
> A series of physical examinations and questions will enable ayurvedic practitioners to discern your dominant *doshas*.

cleansing foods such as kichari (made from basmati rice, mung beans and vegetables) are recommended. Herbal supplements are given to cleanse the bowel and flush out toxins from the liver, blood, sweat glands and skin. These will be specifically designed according to your *dosha* balance. You may be given a massage with herbal oils, heat treatment to open the circulatory channels, and enemas.

Nasya
Otherwise known as nose cleansing, this is part of ayurvedic detoxing that many people have heard of. It involves flushing a medicated oil through the nose and sinuses, in one nostril and out the other, to cleanse toxins from the head and neck. Results can be marked for those who suffer from headaches and migraine, nasal allergies, sinusitis, poor memory or eyesight, and certain neurological conditions.

Benefits
Recent tests of ayurvedic detoxing at the University of Colorado found that those who had undergone several detoxes had significantly lower levels of PCBs, DDT and pesticide residues than the control group. It appeared to be particularly effective on fat-soluble toxins of the kind associated with hormone disruption, suppression of the immune system, allergies, and diseases of the liver and skin. If there is a good ayurvedic clinic near you, it could be worth doing an ayurvedic detox. Some complementary chemists stock well-known ayurvedic remedies that they can recommend to treat individual symptoms, but a complete Panchakarma detox must be done under professional supervision.

Detoxifying massage techniques

There are dozens of different kinds of massage, but the following can be used specifically to enhance the effects of a detox programme.

Manual lymphatic drainage

In the 1930s, Dr Emil Vodder created this technique to stimulate the lymphatic system and help it to eliminate toxins in the cells. MLD is an advanced massage therapy in which the therapist uses special rhythmic pumping techniques to move the skin in the direction of the flow of lymph back to the lymph nodes. It can be used to treat lymphedema (swelling due to fluid accumulation in the tissues), cellulite, sinusitis and arthritis, and it can help to encourage healing after surgery. It's a very pleasant type of massage treatment that would be a useful addition to any detox programme, although it may take several sessions before you see results.

Hot stone therapy

This is a type of massage that uses heated volcanic lava stones. The theory is that their heat helps to increase heart rate and stimulate circulation, thus helping to flush the muscles of toxic waste products. Hot stone therapy is also used to treat depression, stress, PMS, stiff joints and certain skin disorders. In one version of the treatment, you lie on the heated stones and are given a massage with aromatherapy oils. In another form of the therapy, the stones themselves are used to massage your arms, legs and back. Sometimes cold stones are used as well, to further stimulate circulation. The treatment is very relaxing and promotes restful sleep.

> **must know**
>
> **Naturopathy**
> Naturopaths take a broad, holistic view of health and can recommend treatments across a number of different therapies. They will advise on diet, supplements and herbs, exercise and physical therapies, and can also offer psychological support techniques such as counselling. To learn more or find a therapist, see page 149.

Choosing a therapy

6 Holistic detox therapies

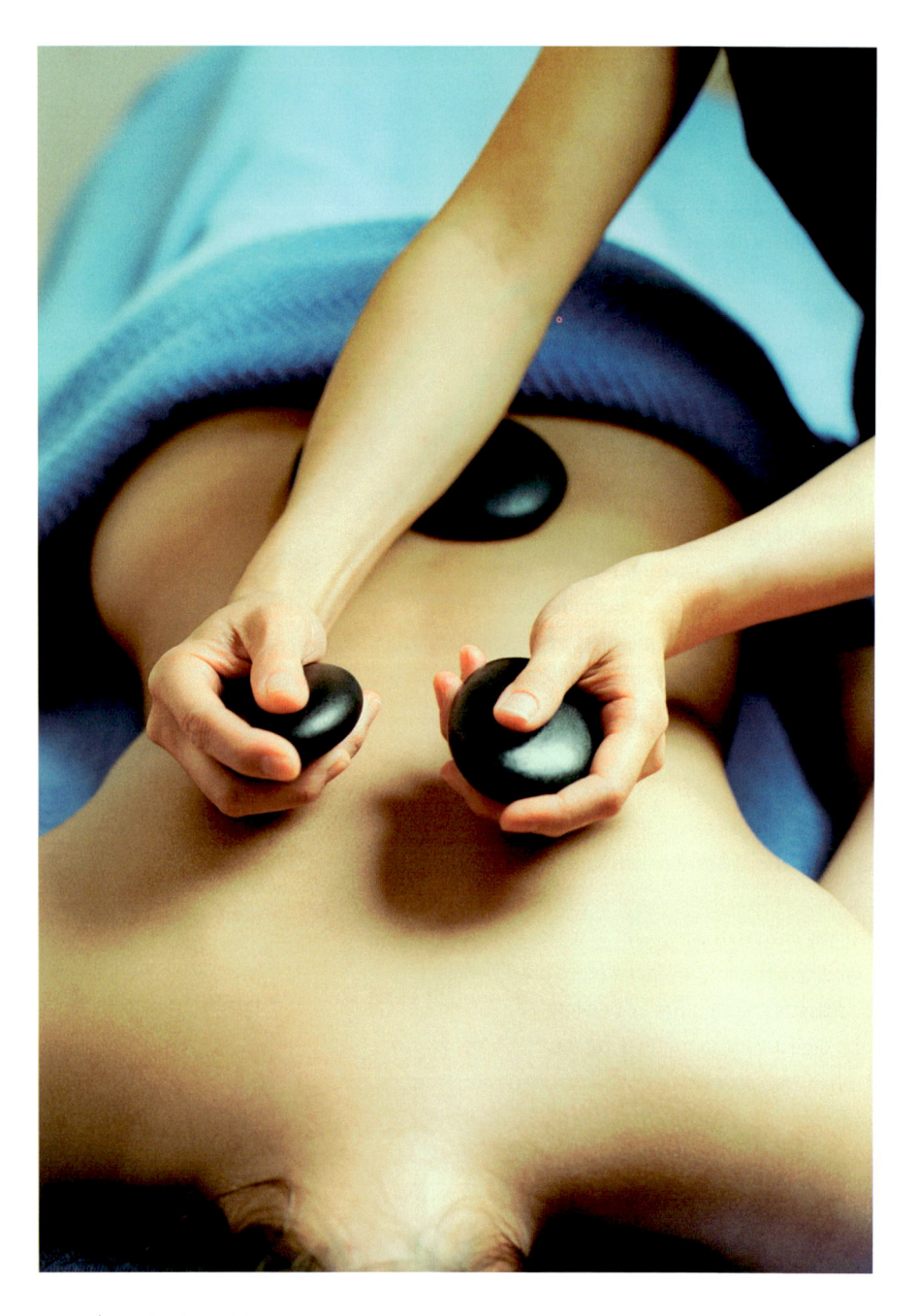

Rolfing

This kind of deep tissue massage was developed by American biochemist Dr Ida P. Rolf in the 1930s. Practitioners are trained to feel for imbalances in the quality, texture and temperature of tissues and thus determine how to reintegrate the body, 'bringing physical balance in the gravitational field'. Rolfing therapists work on your body using hands, fingers, knuckles and even elbows, and the experience can be uncomfortable at times, but it could be worth trying as part of your detox.

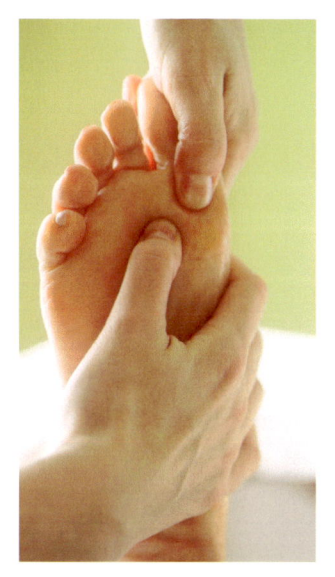

Shiatsu massage

The aim of Shiatsu massage is to balance the flow of *chi* energy along the meridians, and practitioners apply pressure to the same acupoints that are used in acupuncture. Some people report a 'healing crisis' after treatments, such as a headache or flu-like symptoms that last up to 24 hours. These are seen as positive signs that toxins and pent-up emotions are being released. The number of follow-up sessions recommended will vary according to the toxicity of your system.

Reflexology is a method of applying pressure to different parts of the feet to treat a wide range of health problems.

Swedish massage

Swedish massage therapists manipulate muscles and tissues to stimulate the circulatory, nervous and digestive systems and ease stiffness. They believe that emotional tension from past traumas is stored within the muscles and part of their role is to try and release it. Swedish massage can be very effective for treating stress-related conditions, depression, insomnia, digestive disorders such as IBS, and premenstrual syndrome.

Opposite: Stone therapy is now a popular massage technique, which is offered at many health farms and spas.

6 Holistic detox therapies

Reiki

Reiki is a system of healing developed by Japanese theologian Mikao Usui, in which the practitioner makes himself into a channel through which energy flows into the patient to heal their imbalances.

You lie fully clothed on a couch while the therapist places his hands in a sequence of positions that cover the whole body. When you are detoxing, reiki can support and encourage positive personal change such as improving the diet or getting more exercise, and it may reduce cravings for alcohol and tobacco. Is it worth a try? Why not!

Reiki is said to release blockages in the flow of *chi* in the blood.

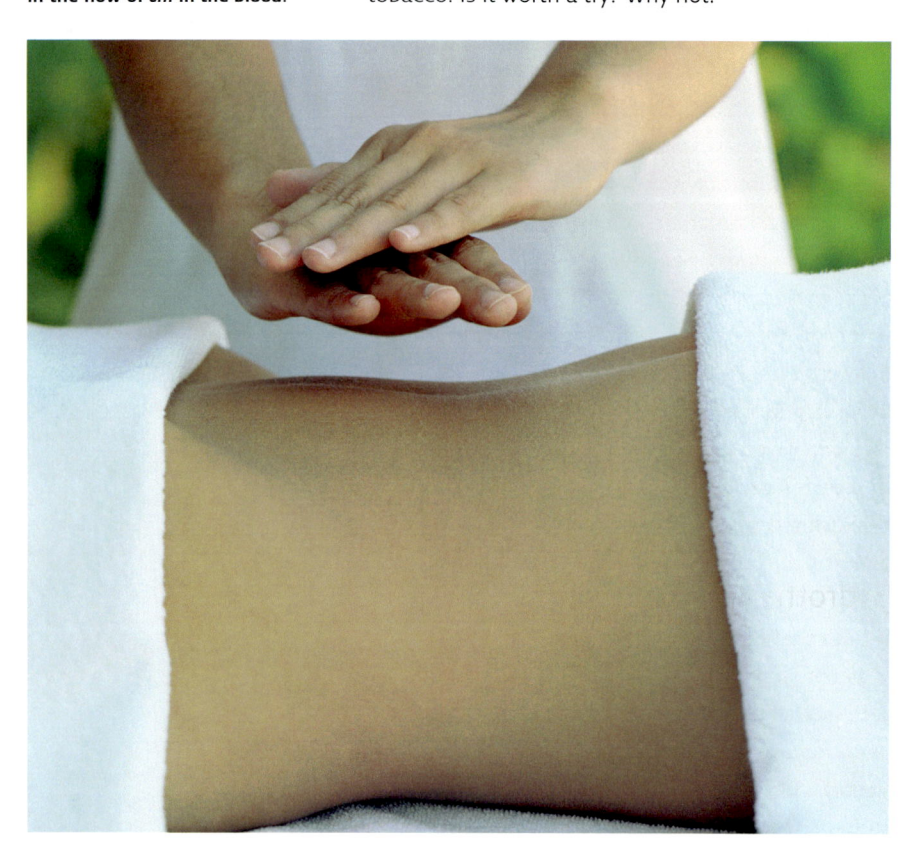

Osteopathy

Osteopathy is a manipulation therapy which reduces strain placed on the body from physical causes such as bad posture or injury, and emotional causes such as stress, anxiety and fear. It can help to relieve digestive disorders such as constipation, hormonal imbalances causing menstrual pain, headaches, insomnia and depression, among other things. If you tell an osteopath that you are detoxing, they can palpate your liver to stimulate its action and support its efforts.

Craniotherapy

Many osteopaths also use craniosacral therapy, or craniotherapy techniques. The brain and spinal cord are surrounded by cerebrospinal fluid that flows up and down with a steady rhythm when we are well. The osteopath is trained to detect tiny variations in the movement of this fluid that indicate emotional or physical trauma in the bones, organs or areas of the body supplied by spinal nerves at each point.

While you lie on your back, the therapist will place their fingers alongside your spine, moving up it, vertebra by vertebra, to feel the place or places where the flow is restricted and they can then free it up using gentle pressure.

Hydrotherapy

This blanket term is now used to refer to all kinds of water-based treatments. Overleaf you will find descriptions of the different hydrotherapy methods that can be particularly useful when you are on a detox programme. The choice is down to personal preference as they are all pleasant and effective.

> **must know**
>
> **The effects of craniotherapy**
> Craniotherapy has a deeply relaxing effect on people and can improve the function of the immune, digestive, respiratory, hormonal and circulatory systems. Some people experience a healing crisis during the 24 hours after their treatment but it should not be too serious. This gentle therapy tends to be highly recommended by all who try it.

6 Holistic detox therapies

> **must know**
>
> **Oral hygiene**
> Keeping your mouth free of bacteria is extremely important. The bacteria that build up can cause tooth decay, receding gums and even heart disease. Buy one of the new sonic toothbrushes that remove much more plaque than manual ones, and always floss and scrape your tongue as well. During a detox, visit a dental hygienist for a thorough clean.

Opposite: During a seaweed wrap, paste is applied to your body to draw out the toxins.

The Kneipp Method

A nineteenth-century Bavarian monk, Father Sebastian Kneipp, invented this technique which claims to cure illness by helping the body to get rid of its waste products. It uses a programme of hot and cold baths, steam baths and herbal wraps to cleanse and detoxify, improve the circulation, stimulate the flow of lymph and help the digestive system.

A therapist will talk to you first and will design a programme to suit your specific problems, but the elements could include one or some of the following:
• A hot herbal bath with lavender and rosemary, and possibly some salts and oils as well.
• A moor bath, which is a hot, muddy sludge of herbs in which you relax for up to 20 minutes.
• High-powered jets of hot or cold water directed onto your back to stimulate the circulation.
• Sitz baths, one filled with hot and one with cold water, which are used as a circulation stimulator. You stand with your feet in the hot water until they are warmed through, then you step into the cold water until they cool down, and repeat several times. Salts may be added to the water to intensify the detoxifying effects.
• A herbal wrap in which you lie with herbs bound tightly around you to make you sweat and draw out impurities through the pores.
• Water-based sessions may be followed by a Swedish massage.

Thalassotherapy

Popular at many spa resorts, this term comes from the Greek word *thalassos*, meaning sea, and is used for any treatment involving seawater or seaweed.

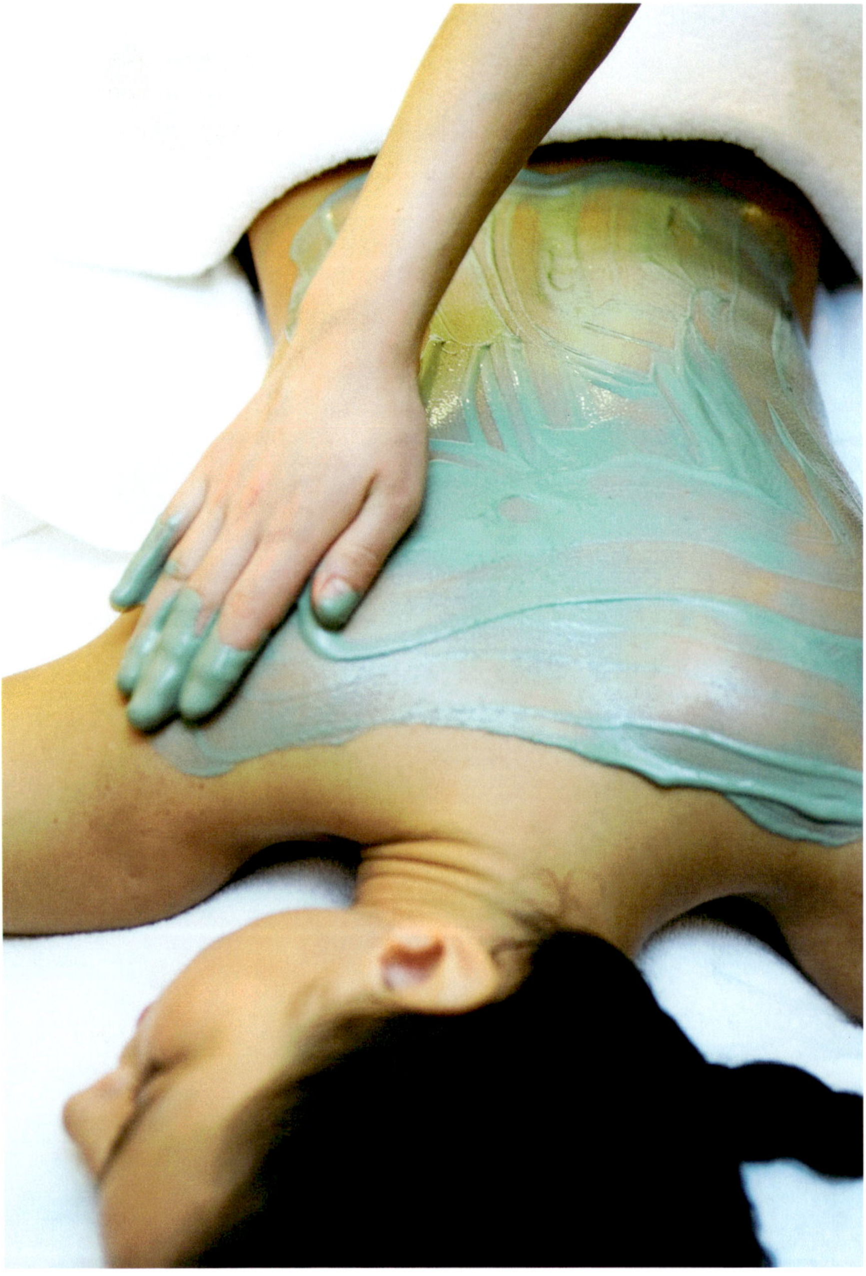

6 Holistic detox therapies

> **must know**
>
> **Finding therapists**
> To find a clinic offering the therapies described in this chapter, check your local directory or surf the internet. Many complementary health clinics offer a wide range of treatments, and you can be cross-referred between therapists. To find a spa holiday, ask your travel agent or look on the net!

Jacuzzis, whether with seawater or not, are now one of the most relaxing therapies on offer at spas, and many local gyms now have them, too.

Seawater is rich in minerals which are great for drawing out toxins, cleansing and toning the skin, so many thalassotherapy treatments involve swimming in a heated seawater pool or being pummelled with jets of seawater.

Seaweed wraps
These are a very popular technique, and are said to boost the circulation, stimulate the metabolism

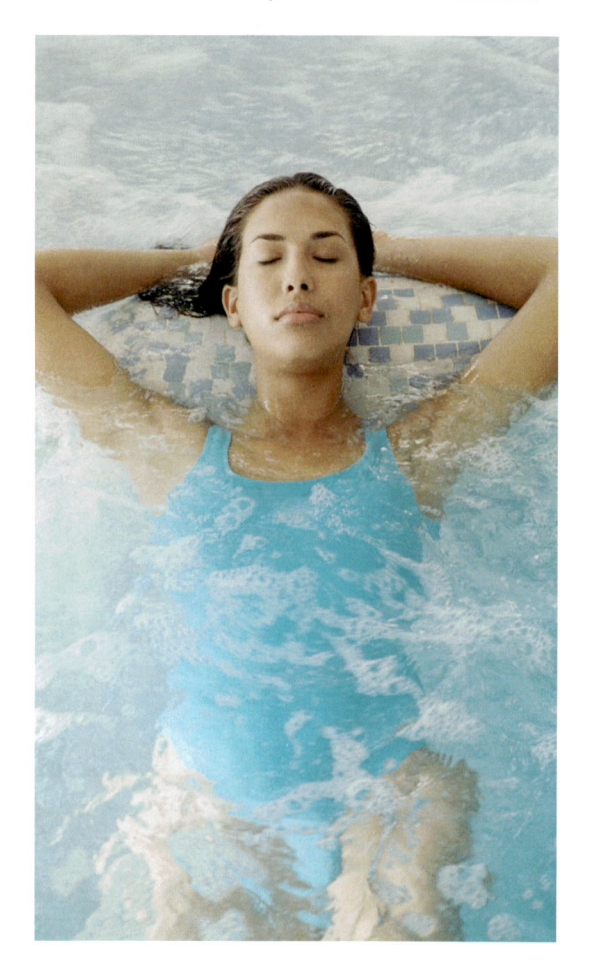

and encourage the elimination of toxins. They are particularly recommended for treating cellulite, sagging skin and stretch marks, and some people even claim to lose a few centimetres after a wrap. What generally happens is that a trained therapist will smooth seaweed paste all over your body, targeting specific areas if you wish. You are wrapped in warm thermal sheets and then left for up to 45 minutes, after which you shower it all off. It is important to drink extra water after a seaweed wrap so that you do not become dehydrated.

Thalassotherapy treatments are incredibly relaxing and most people will notice a great improvement in both their skin texture and tone after one of these treatments.

Saunas and steam baths

Many local gyms now offer saunas (a hot dry room) or steam baths (hot and steamy) to help eliminate impurities through sweating. However, don't overdo it. Start with a five-minute sauna or steam and do not ever spend more than 20 minutes in there or you could feel very dizzy and unwell.

Resist the temptation to keep throwing extra water on a sauna's coals to increase the heat. Those people with high blood pressure, heart disease, asthma or epilepsy should avoid saunas or steam baths, as they could exacerbate your condition.

Some people use a spatula to scrape off the sweat and released toxins. Alternatively, you can have a good rub-down with a loofah or brush in the shower afterwards to slough off any dead skin cells as well as waste products. Do as the Swedes do and follow up with a stimulating cold shower afterwards.

want to know more?

• Read Ian Belcher's entertaining description of a detox holiday in Koh Samui, complete with graphic details, at: www.guardian.co.uk/weekend/story/0,3605,663391,00.html.

weblinks

• To find an acupuncturist contact the British Acupuncture Council on: tel: 020 8735 0400 www.acupuncture.org.uk
• To find a naturopath, contact the College of Naturopathic Medicine: tel: 01342 410505 www.naturopathy.uk.com
• To find an ayurvedic practitioner, contact Ayurveda UK on: tel: 01283 815669 www.ayurveda.uk.com
• For a listing of the complementary health practitioners in each region, log on to: www.chisuk.org.uk/directory

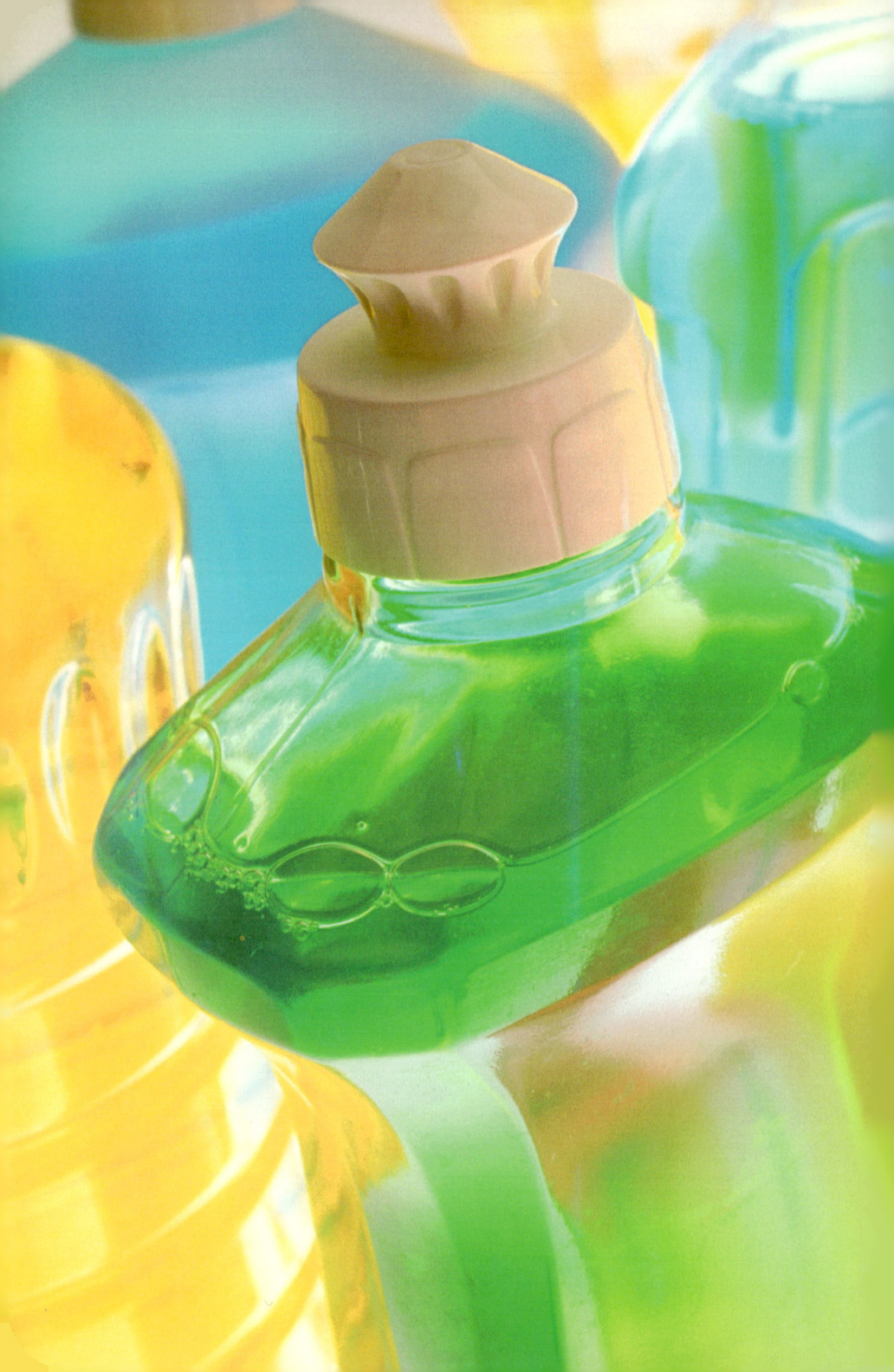

7 Toxins that surround us

You have cleared your diet of artificial additives and are encouraging your body to detoxify, yet as you sit reading this book there are toxins all around you. They could be in the toothpaste and antiperspirant you used this morning, in the furniture you are sitting on, the carpet under your feet, and the cleaning products, paints and varnishes you have used all over your home. In the garden, they are in the pesticides that stop slugs eating your plants as well as the creosote on the fence. You may not be able to do much about the toxins in the air you breathe – but for all the rest, there are safer alternatives.

7 Toxins that surround us

Everyday toxins

Beware! Reading this chapter and finding out about all the nasty substances in the products you use daily will almost certainly change your shopping habits forever!

must know

Animal testing
If you are against animal testing, you should be aware that when a label says a product is 'not tested on animals', it can simply mean that although the whole product was not tested on animals, several of the key ingredients may have been.

Playing with chemistry

Twentieth-century chemists were extremely proud of themselves when they invented brand-new chemical compounds that could dissolve even the toughest dried-in grease in our ovens, make our laundry whiter-than-white, penetrate and plump out ageing skin cells, kill all known germs, and keep us odour-free all day long. Synthetic materials, like rayon and nylon, were all the rage, carpets were treated to make them virtually indestructible, and timber was sealed so that it would never rot. Alternatively, you could buy brand-new particleboard products made of wood fibre and held together with synthetic resin. Life was getting better and better for us all – or was it?

None of these products make you keel over gasping and wheezing on first exposure (except perhaps the oven cleaner) but the toxins they contain have a cumulative effect with long-term exposure that scientists are still investigating today. They are only now finding out that cosmetics and personal care items containing parabens seem to be linked to breast cancer – although it is hardly surprising, since parabens mimic the action of oestrogen in the body. It was long thought that mercury could not leach out of fillings once they were in place, but autopsies are finding a direct correlation between the amount of mercury in the brain cells and the number of fillings that a person has in their teeth.

Dry-cleaning solvents containing perchloroethylene (perc, for short) are excellent at removing stains without damaging the fabric, but they have now been linked to cancer, liver and nervous system damage, infertility and hormone disruption.

What is 'natural'?

Maybe it is time to cut the chemistry and go back to nature in our quest for good health. But what does 'natural' mean? The truth is that it is virtually meaningless when used on a product label. By law, only a small percentage of the ingredients need to be 'natural' for this term to be used.

You will find some confusing phrases used on packaging. The term 'derived from natural coconut oil', for example, can actually refer to cocamide DEA, a foaming agent used in some shampoos, which is extracted from coconut oil by the addition of a solvent known as diethanolanine, which is widely thought to be carcinogenic.

What is 'organic'?

Can you trust the term 'organic'? Some manufacturers have played with the word in the past, for example claiming to use 'organic herbs' in a product that is otherwise entirely composed of synthetic chemicals. In theory, the unscrupulous could even claim that a toxic petrochemical preservative, such as methyl parabens, is organic, because it comes from leaves that rotted thousands of years ago to become crude oil, which was then used to make this preservative.

must know

Alternatives to dry cleaning

Greenpeace believes that the best option currently available is wet cleaning, a process in which garments are immersed in water and eco-friendly detergents, then carefully dried and stretched back into shape. However, this will cause more fabric deterioration than dry cleaning. If you decide to dry clean a garment, hang it outdoors to air for as long as possible afterwards, so that the toxic residues can evaporate.

7 Toxins that surround us

But, in fact, the organic market is controlled very carefully. Organic standards boards only grant organic status to those products that pass stringent testing procedures. To be on the safe side, look out for organic kitemarks and certification if a product claims to be organic. The companies recommended in this chapter are all trustworthy.

Personal grooming

Toxins are eliminated through the skin via perspiration but they can also be absorbed through the skin via hair follicles and sebaceous glands (although not through sweat glands). You will not ever hear skincare manufacturers claiming that their products penetrate through the skin and into the blood circulation, because they would then be classified as drugs and subject to much more

Avoid those 'antiperspirants' that prevent sweating altogether; opt for 'deodorants' that allow your body to shed the toxins in sweat but prevent it smelling bad.

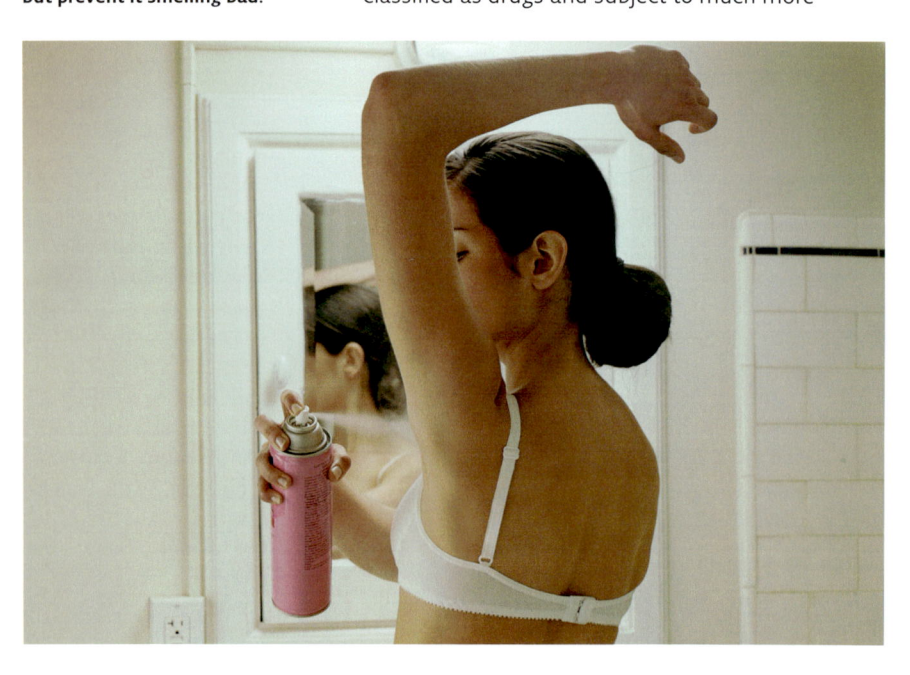

stringent testing and regulation. However, there is plenty of evidence that skin does absorb some ingredients from skincare preparations because they are turning up in our blood, urine, organs and tissues. Scientists often find phthalates in urine, parabens in breast tumours, and synthetic fragrances like musk xylene in human fat.

It is ironic that cosmetic companies pour so much research funding into the development of new products that help to disguise the signs of ageing (anti-wrinkle creams, hair-thickening shampoos and conditioners, firming body lotions) yet they use ingredients that some researchers suspect of being carcinogens, neurological toxins, immune suppressants and hormone disruptors, so the net effect can be drastically ageing!

In the US, the Environmental Working Group tested 120 cosmetic products, including shampoos, moisturizers, foundations and lip balm, and found ingredients certified by the US Government as 'known or probable carcinogens' in each and every one. In 2005, the US Food and Drug Administration declared that consumers should be informed of the fact that many commercial shampoos, deodorants, perfumes, nail polishes, hand creams, hair dyes and bubble baths have not been safety tested, despite the fact that they commonly contain chemicals that disrupt the hormones, are carcinogenic and disrupt the nervous system. Here are some examples.

Phthalates

These are solvents found in fragrance and nail polish, as well as a substance added to plastics to make them more flexible. They have been linked to

must know

Deodorants
To avoid parabens and aluminium salts, opt for alum crystal deodorants. They don't block the sweat glands but they inhibit bacterial growth in your sweat, which is what causes the odour. They are available in spray, roll-on, cream or the original crystallized rock form from chemists or the organic websites listed on page 190.

7 Toxins that surround us

liver and thyroid damage, cancer, low sperm counts in men, miscarriages and birth defects. They are not easy to avoid, however, because they will not be listed on the ingredients label.

Parabens
Parabens (methyl, propyl and butyl) have all been linked to breast cancer (which can affect men as well as women, although less commonly) and they can also cause contact skin rashes.

DEA-related compounds
Topical application of DEA-related compounds (cocamide, lauramide and myristamide) has been linked to cancer by some experts.

Ceteareth-12
An emulsifier called Ceteareth-12 may contain dangerous levels of carcinogenic ethylene oxide and dioxane.

Antiperspirants
These often contain aluminium salts that prevent the body from sweating. Aluminium build-up in brain cells has been linked to Alzheimer's disease.

Skin irritants
Many cosmetic additives can be skin irritants, such as lanolin, glycerol and cetyl alcohol, which are found in a wide range of products.

Avoiding harmful chemicals
The best way to steer clear of harmful ingredients is to opt for organic brands of everything you apply to

must know

Allergy help
Allergy UK has a chemical sensitivity division with lots of handy tips and alternatives for those who are allergic to everyday products. For details, see page 190.

your skin, including body- and face-care products, makeup, soaps, sunscreen, toothpaste and all other toiletries. You should be able to find them in large chemists or department stores, or try the websites listed on pages 190-191 (many of them will send you catalogues on request).

Mercury fillings

Most British adults have at least one or two mercury fillings in their mouths, yet research shows that the average-sized filling contains 750,000 micrograms of mercury and releases around 10 micrograms a day. This vapour is inhaled and travels up to the hippocampus of the brain, which controls memory. People with Alzheimer's disease have mercury levels in their brains that are two to three times higher than those who do not. Low-level mercury exposure can damage the brain, heart, lungs, liver, kidneys, thyroid, pituitary, adrenal glands, immune system, and just about every aspect of body function.

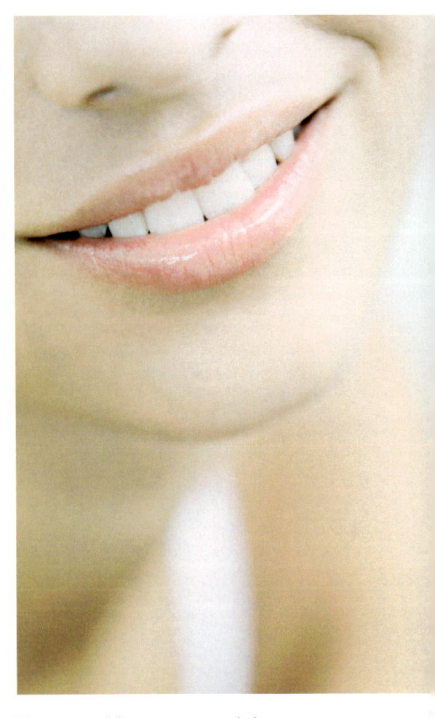

You can whiten your teeth by brushing with bicarbonate of soda; avoid the strong chemicals in whitening toothpastes and bleaching products.

Replacing fillings

Should you rush to have your mercury fillings replaced? Certainly not, say most experts. The process of removing fillings can generate much more mercury vapour as well as stray particles as your dentist drills into them with a high-speed drill. If you are worried that your fillings are damaging your health, find a specialist who will test your urine for heavy metal content. If your levels are high, seek out a dentist who specializes in amalgam removal and only have one or two fillings replaced at a time. A rubber dam should be used to prevent you swallowing any particles and a high-speed suction

7 Toxins that surround us

You may have to use a little more elbow grease when you throw out your toxic cleaning products.

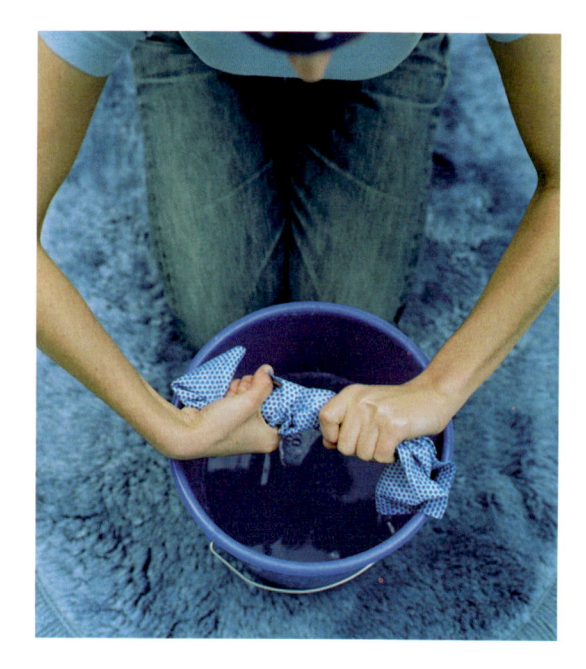

must know

A cleaner home?
Over the past 20 years, our consumption of household cleaning products has risen sharply in the UK, and there is a corresponding rise in the level of VOCs (volatile organic compounds) in the atmosphere. These can cause irritation of the airways when present in low concentrations and, according to a 2003 study, may increase the risk of childhood asthma.

device should be in your mouth at all times. You may also be given a nose mask to stop you inhaling mercury vapour (if it is not offered, then ask for one). Some experts recommend that you undergo chelation therapy after filling removal to rid your system of any ingested mercury. If you ask your dentist, they will probably recommend that it's safer to leave mercury fillings in than take them out. Obviously, if a filling breaks or falls out anyway, that is the time to replace it with a safer (and more attractive) white alternative.

Household cleaning products
In the US, 12 per cent of emergency calls to the Poison Control Center are due to people ingesting household cleaning products. The damage they do if you accidentally swallow them is very clear, but

it is less obvious what's happening when we inhale them or absorb ingredients through our skin. You will probably want to avoid products that contain the following substances.

Chlorine bleaches

These are found in toilet cleaners, washing powders and dishwasher detergents, and they can create carcinogenic substances when broken down. If they come into contact with products containing ammonia, a gas called chloramine is formed that can cause severe respiratory reactions.

Optical brighteners

These give the illusion of whiteness by attaching themselves to fabrics and reflecting bright light but they can cause severe skin irritation.

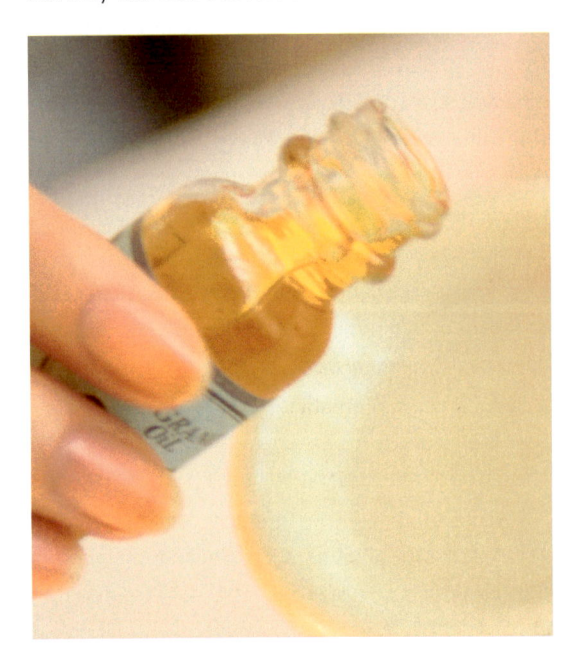

must know

Eco-balls
These chemical-free laundry balls work by producing ionized oxygen, activating the water molecules to penetrate the fabrics and lift away dirt. They are hypo-allergenic and leave no residues behind, and each one lasts for 750 washes.

Add frankincense oil to an aromatherapy burner and inhale to help rebuild your energy levels and freshen the air in your home.

7 Toxins that surround us

must know

Chemical sensitivity
The British Society for Allergy, Environmental and Nutritional Medicine has been urging the UK government to tighten the regulations on testing of existing and new chemicals. They are finding evidence of a syndrome called 'multiple chemical sensitivity', in which sufferers develop a severe allergy to everyday chemicals even in minute doses. According to the European Chemicals Bureau, only 14 per cent of the most heavily used chemicals have a full set of safety data available to the public. That means we don't know the long-term effects of most of the chemicals we use in our homes.

Butyl cellulose
This is found in heavy-duty all-purpose cleaners and can be absorbed through the skin and lungs. Some experts think it causes liver and kidney damage. At low levels, it may be responsible for headaches, dizziness, nausea and fainting.

Anionic surfactants
These are present in some cleaners and can be contaminated with carcinogenic nitrosamines.

Carpet cleaners
These often contain butyl cellulose (see above) and may also contain perchloroethylene (the dry cleaning fluid, see page 153).

Phosphates
These are used in washing powder to improve cleaning and soften the water but they pollute our waterways by encouraging the growth of algae that starve the water of oxygen, killing fish and plant life.

Oven cleaners and metal polishes
Oven cleaners may contain 'lye', which gives off toxic fumes that can burn the skin and eyes. Metal polishes contain petroleum products that can damage the nervous system, kidneys and eyes.

Avoiding toxins
The list goes on! To avoid any toxic nasties, always choose a reputable organic brand in the supermarket, or buy your cleaning products from a reputable organic source (see page 189). You might also want to consider using some old-fashioned natural

Natural cleaning

- Use vinegar in warm water to clean work surfaces, chrome, mirrors and glass.
- Polish furniture with beeswax mixed with a little lemon essential oil.
- Freshen the air with your choice of aromatherapy oil in a sprayer full of water.
- Clean your oven with bicarbonate of soda, hot water and stainless steel wool.
- Choose laundry soap instead of detergents and add half a cup of washing soda as a softener.
- Bleach white clothes in sunlight, or add soda crystals to your wash.
- To descale your kettle, cover the element with equal quantities of vinegar and water, bring to the boil and leave to soak overnight before scrubbing clean.
- To clean the toilet bowl, mix a paste of borax and lemon juice and leave for 20 minutes before scrubbing.
- For an effective cleaner for the bath, basin and tiles, mix baking soda, white vinegar, lemon essential oil and tea tree oil.
- To clean carpets or rugs, mix warm water, organic liquid soap, 1 tsp borax and a splash of vinegar. Sponge on, leave to dry and vacuum off.

cleansing solutions (see above). They are often more effective than their modern chemical equivalents.

In the home

You have probably heard about the risks associated with paints, paint strippers, fuels, glues and permanent markers that contain volatile organic compounds (VOCs). The fumes from these can cause nausea, headaches and drowsiness, and prolonged exposure has been linked with cancer. Next time you decide to redecorate your home, make sure that you choose organic, water-based paints, stains, sealants, thinners and markers, which emit only natural, pleasant fragrances.

7 Toxins that surround us

must know

Sanitary protection
Nearly all the major-brand tampons contain a mixture of rayon, which creates an ideal environment for the staphylococcus bacteria that causes toxic shock syndrome, as well as conventionally grown cotton, which has been exposed to many kinds of pesticides and fertilizers. Some of the chemicals used to bleach tampons have been implicated in the formation of dioxin, which can harm the inside of the vagina and may be linked to endometriosis. Choose organic tampons or pads.

Carpets and cushions

Many carpets are treated with pesticides, fungicides and dyes that can give off vapours that we inhale or chemicals that can be absorbed through the skin. The latex backing used on 95 per cent of carpets contains styrene, a suspected carcinogen, and carpets can also contain volatile organic compounds and formaldehyde, low levels of which can irritate the eyes, nose and throat. The adhesive used for office carpets, known as 4-phenylcyclohexene (4-PC), is thought to contribute to 'sick building syndrome'. The healthiest carpets are hessian-backed and not treated with pesticides; choose organic wool cotton or hemp without biocides (to deter mould) or stain protectors.

Watch out for polyurethane stuffing in sofa cushions, as some experts think it can give off toxic chemicals that you inhale while watching TV. Ideally, cushions should be stuffed with cotton or wool, but polyester fill is your next best option.

Woods

Synthetic urea formaldehyde resin is often used in manufactured woods (like MDF, particleboard or chipboard). Fumes continue to leak from these products for years, so it is best that you avoid manufactured woods.

However, some timber treatments can also be toxic, containing lindane (now banned, but could be found on older wood products and is linked to breast cancer), PCP (an organochlorine fungicide) and other insecticides and colourings. Opt instead for organic wood which has been treated with natural chemicals like beeswax and borax.

Fabrics

We spend hours every night surrounded by bed linen, and during the daylight hours our skin is in constant contact with our clothes, so it makes sense to think about the chemicals that are used in the manufacture of fabrics.

Synthetic fabrics, such as nylon and rayon, are produced using a wide range of chemicals, and more than 35 different herbicides and pesticides are used in the growing of conventional cotton crops. If you want to avoid these, you should opt for organic cotton or hemp, which is grown without the use of any man-made chemicals. All the dyes are plant or mineral based, and no heavy metals or harmful chemicals are used in the dyeing or finishing processes of these natural organic fabrics.

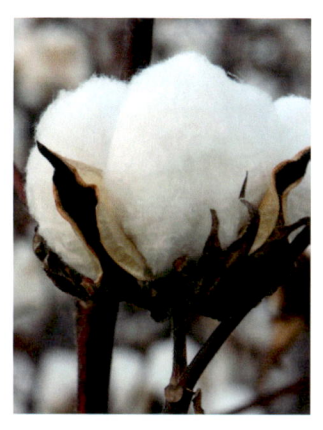

Around 40 per cent of cotton grown in the USA is genetically modified; huge amounts of agro-chemicals are used on the crops.

Fires

Finally, it is important to make sure that any oil or gas fires are checked regularly by a qualified engineer to ensure they are functioning correctly and are not slowly poisoning you when in use. It is less common nowadays but you still read in the newspapers about cases of people dying in their sleep while a faulty heater pumped out carbon monoxide into the atmosphere.

Insecticides

None of us want our homes to be overrun by ants, our clothes to be eaten by moths or our barbecues to be ruined by a plague of mosquitoes but, when you think about it, sprays or powders that cause insects to drop dead in their tracks cannot be doing us much good either.

must know

Mattresses
The wool used to stuff mattresses is often chemically treated and research shows that these chemicals can emit vapours that we breathe in as we sleep. Cover your mattress with a cotton barrier cloth or buy a new, organic one. You should also avoid plastic sheets (such as those used when children are being potty-trained), as the plastic can give off harmful emissions.

Everyday toxins | 163

7 Toxins that surround us

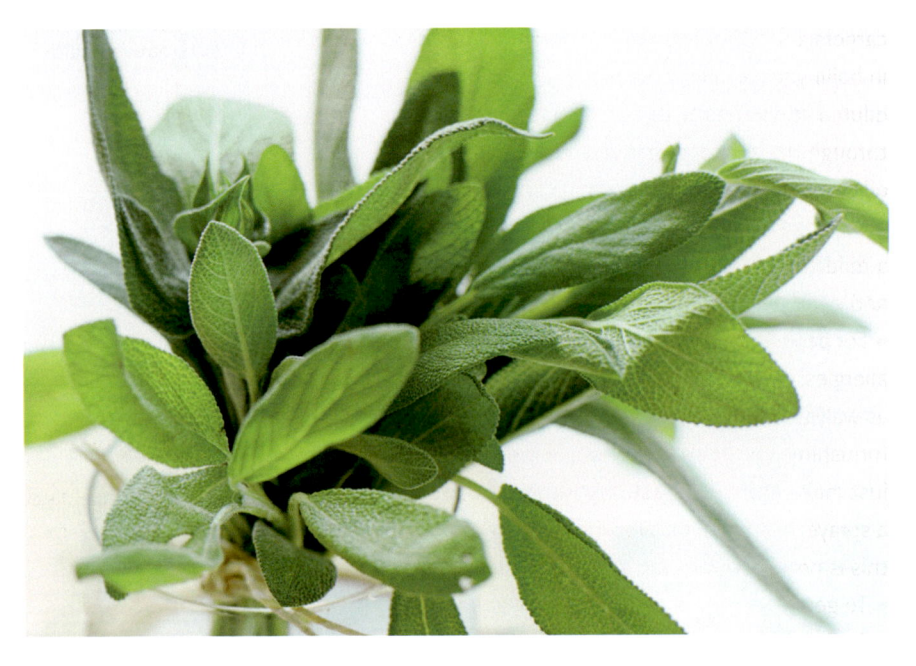

Sage repels all kinds of insects.

Non-toxic bug control

Fortunately, there are plenty of natural, non-toxic ways of dealing with common bugs in the home and garden. Try the following and see for yourself.

- The herb tansy, planted in the garden, will deter ants. Indoors, pile dried mint, chilli powder or borax at strategic points.
- Finely ground eggshells deter slugs in the garden and act as a fertilizer as well.
- Cockroaches, moths and rodents all hate sage, so tie bunches round the home.
- Burn citronella candles to deter mosquitoes when you're sitting outside on a summer evening.
- Instead of mothballs, use pieces of muslin soaked in cedarwood, camphor or lavender oil and placed around the house, especially in wardrobes.
- If your cat or dog brings home fleas, vacuum the

carpets and soft furnishings and wash what you can in boiling water. Spray tea tree and eucalyptus oils diluted in water onto furniture and carpets. Comb through the animal's coat with a mixture of olive oil, mint, eucalyptus and tea tree oil, squashing or drowning fleas you comb out, then shampoo with a mild baby shampoo with a few drops of tea tree and eucalyptus mixed in.

• For people with asthma associated with dust mite allergies, it's best to remove their homes, such as wall-to-wall carpets and over-stuffed soft furnishings. To neutralize dust mites in these areas, just make a cup of very strong black tea, put it in a sprayer and spray on problem areas. (Obviously, this is not ideal on cream sofas!)

• To get rid of aphids (e.g. greenfly and blackfly), spider mites and scale mites, steep two garlic cloves in a litre of water for 24 hours, then spray all over the affected plants.

• Is there an ants' nest in your garden? If so, just

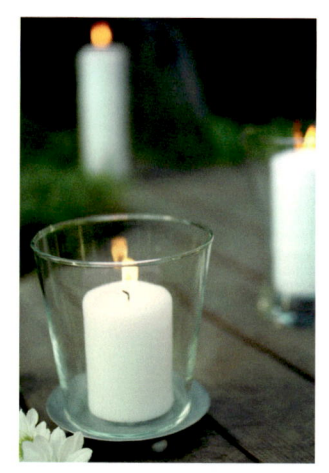

Scented garden candles can deter insects and produce attractive flickering light as well.

must know

Headlice
If your child comes home from school with headlice, do not buy the over-the-counter treatments containing malathione, a strong chemical that is rapidly absorbed into the tissues. Blend some lavender, tea tree and eucalyptus oils in warmed olive oil and apply all over the child's hair. Leave overnight, then comb through with a fine-toothed nit comb and rinse off. A drop of tea tree oil in hair conditioner two or three times a week is a good preventive measure.

7 Toxins that surround us

Your lungs need to be in good shape to filter the oxygen we need to stay alive from the other toxic fumes in our atmosphere.

pour boiling water over them. Pure lemon juice works as well but it's better to save it for use in detox drinks and recipes.

- To keep wasps away from a picnic or any outdoor meal, half-fill a tumbler with fruit juice and secure a paper lid over the top – hold it in place with a rubber band. Pierce a hole through the paper with a pencil. Wasps will crawl through, attracted by the scent of the juice, but will not be able to get out again.

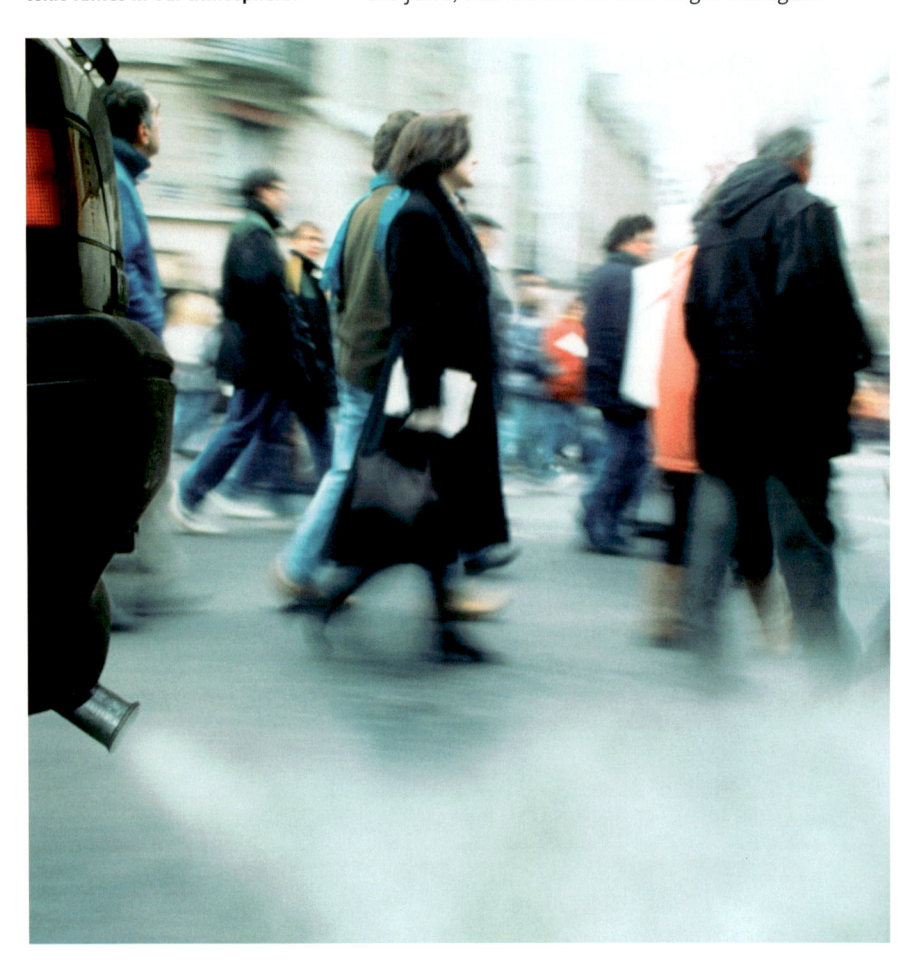

The air we breathe

When you are in an area with a lot of traffic, you know all about it. The air smells poisonous – and it is. Traffic emissions contain benzene (linked to leukaemia), carbon monoxide (makes you tired, causes memory loss, can cause chest pain and miscarriage), diesel particles (linked to circulatory disease and lung cancer), petrol (may damage the nervous system and lungs), polycyclic aromatic hydrocarbons (linked to reproductive problems and cancer) and total petroleum hydrocarbons (which may affect the circulatory and immune systems, the skin, lungs and eyes). You are breathing in even more of these chemicals while sitting in your car than out in the street, because the air pumped in for heating and air conditioning systems is at ground level where the exhaust fumes are pumped out.

Do you think that you would be better off moving to the country instead? Well, the air there can be full of agricultural pesticides and fertilizers. These contain carbamates (which some experts think disrupt the nervous system and can cause rashes and fatigue at low levels), organochlorines (which are thought to build up in the fat cells and over the long term can cause weakness and tremors), organophosphates (high levels are fatal and low levels are linked to skin rashes and fatigue) and pyrethroids (linked to nervous system damage and respiratory system irritation).

Should you just stay indoors? Well, according to the Environmental Protection Agency in the US, indoor air can be two to five times more polluted than outdoors. So you can't win, or can you?

> **must know**
>
> **Cooking warnings**
> Avoid non-stick pans that are coated in perfluorooctanioic acids (PFOAs), which are subsequently found in foods cooked in them. Avoid polyethylene terephthalate (PET) plastic containers for heating foods in a microwave or storing wet foods or acidic liquids, such as wine or juice. Avoid boil-in-the-bag foods, because of the risk of antimony leaking from the plastic. Smoking cooking oils or charred meats, e.g. on barbecues, can both be carcinogenic to inhale and to eat, so don't have the heat too high.

7 Toxins that surround us

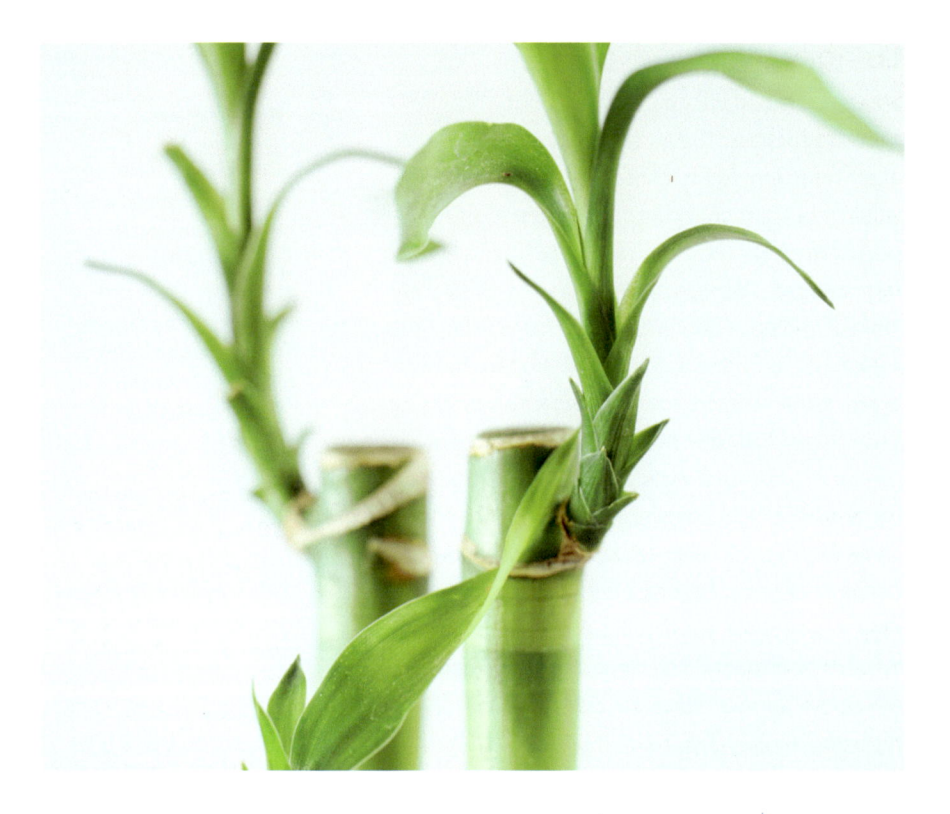

Fill your home and office with green plants to absorb toxins and to boost oxygen. Bamboo is especially good for this.

must know

Radon
Here's one more thing to worry about! Radon is a radioactive gas formed from the breakdown of uranium in the earth and it is more common in areas that have a lot of granite and limestone in the topsoil. Breathing in tiny particles of radon can increase your chance of getting lung cancer, but there are measures that can reduce your risk level. Contact your environmental health officer, or look at the Health Protection Agency's website at: www.hpa.org.uk/radiation/radar/index.htm.

Combatting the problem

So what can you do, given that the average human needs to breathe between 8,000 and 10,000 litres of air a day to stay alive? Well, you can open the windows and ventilate your house as much as possible. Houseplants can reduce levels of formaldehyde, benzene and other contaminants in the atmosphere as they absorb them as a source of food. Palms, bamboo and peace lilies are particularly good decontaminants.

Outdoors, try to choose routes that are tree-lined, or where there are a lot of plants, because the process of photosynthesis removes some harmful gases from the atmosphere and produces more oxygen. Take particular care when exercising outdoors as you are breathing in huge lungfuls of air and your circulation is speeding it rapidly round your system. Cyclists are advised to wear masks for riding in towns and in the countryside.

Don't panic, however. If you have a respiratory disease, such as asthma or emphysema, you might consider moving to a less polluted part of the country, but airborne toxins are pretty endemic and traces are found in tests on people who live on some of the UK's most remote islands.

Concentrate on avoiding the toxins you can do something about – in the products you buy. Read labels carefully; if there is a long string of complex chemicals, give those products a miss. Choose natural ingredients, such as essential oils, herbs and sea salts, and look for certified organic brands. You can't avoid all the toxins in modern life, but if you try not to ingest them voluntarily, you will be taking a huge step towards looking after your health.

want to know more?

- Allergy UK has a chemical sensitivity division. Call 020 8303 8525 or visit the website: www.allergyuk.org

weblinks

- For research on the effects of chemicals and pesticides, go to: www.chem-tox.com
- For cleaning materials and where to buy them see the following:
www.greenpeople.co.uk
www.SoOrganic.com
www.ecomerchant.co.uk
- Cyclists' masks, see: www.cyclexpress.co.uk/categories/AntiPollution_Masks_677.asp
- For non-toxic paints, varnishes, wood stains: www.ecopaints.co.uk
www.ieko.co.uk
www.earthbornpaints.co.uk
www.greenbuildingstore.co.uk
- For dozens of tips on toxin-free gardening, see: www.organicgardening.co.uk

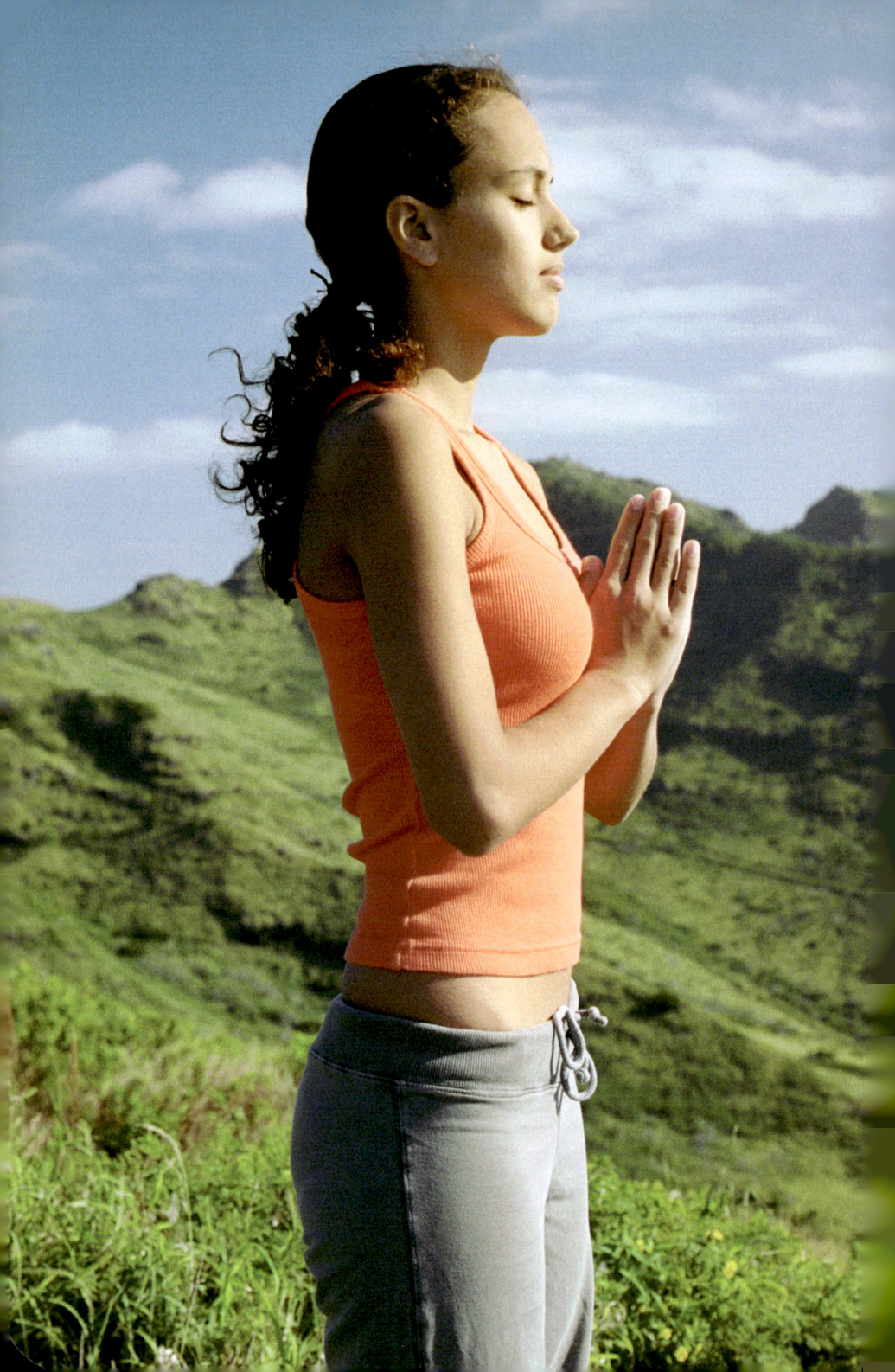

8 Emotional detoxing

It is not just environmental and food toxins that can poison us – we are all familiar with the horrible sensation of negative emotions eating away at our insides. Feelings such as jealousy, resentment, frustration and unexpressed anger can become internal poisons that ultimately damage our wellbeing and quality of life if they're not resolved. More and more scientific trials and studies are finding that a positive outlook and emotional contentment have a beneficial effect on our physical health, while those with a negative view of the world fare less well healthwise. Why not use the time when you are cleansing your body during a detox to try a deep cleanse of your emotions as well?

8 Emotional detoxing

Deep-cleanse your emotional life

Emotional detoxing means getting rid of all those feelings and behaviours that can poison your life and detract from your happiness. Try the exercises in this chapter to identify the toxic parts of your life and think about how you can heal them.

> **must know**
>
> **Depression makes you ill**
> Studies have found that those with depression are at higher risk of heart disease and other illnesses. Researchers at the University of Wisconsin recently proved that the activation of the brain regions associated with negative emotions appears to weaken the immune system response to a flu vaccine.

Who is on your train?

Get a piece of paper and a pen and draw the outline of a train with six carriages. In the front carriage, write the names of the people who are most important in your life. In the second carriage, write the names of those who are next most important. Continue through the carriages, including all the people who play a regular part in your life, whether friends, family or work colleagues. It does not matter how many you put in each carriage, whether it's 10 or just one.

When you have finished, have a look at your train. You may be surprised at who you decided to include in the first carriage. Perhaps you had not consciously considered how much certain people meant to you. Conversely, you may have demoted someone who would expect to be right up there.

A question that takes some people by surprise when they look at their front carriage is: did you put yourself in? If not, why not? Aren't you the most important person in your life? If you're not, you should be. Your relationships with other people are never going to run smoothly if you don't value yourself enough. Put yourself in now, in the middle of the front carriage.

Creating a mind map

For the next part of this exercise, you need a large sheet of paper and a set of coloured pens or pencils. You are going to create something known as a mind map. Start by writing your own name right in the centre of the piece of paper, then write the names of the occupants of the first train carriage around you, like an inner circle of planets orbiting your Sun.

Now draw a line between you and each of these people, choosing a colour for each that somehow represents the state of your relationship – just select the colour that feels right to you. When you've finished linking them to you, draw in the links that join them to each other, where these exist. Your boss might not have a relationship with your mother, but your partner will. Once again, choose the colours that feel right.

When you've finished linking up the occupants of the first carriage, write the names of those in the second carriage, slightly further away but still orbiting around you, and draw in the coloured links, first between you and them, and then between them and all the others. Do the same for the third, fourth, fifth and sixth carriages, drawing a coloured link between each of them and you but omitting the links between each other, unless they are very significant, or your mind map will get too messy.

You probably know what's coming next. Sit back and consider the colours you chose for each link and what you meant when you chose them. Look at the ones that have negative connotations for you, in the inner circle to start off with. Are you angry with that person? Do you fully understand why you are angry with them? Or are you jealous, or hurt, or resentful?

> **must know**
>
> **Feel the fear**
> Emotional detoxing can feel very scary because we fear losing someone as a result. Sometimes this happens and sometimes it doesn't. You need to feel quite strong in yourself to look inside and consider making changes, so make sure you are being nice to yourself at the same time. Augment the positive and don't give yourself a hard time.

8 Emotional detoxing

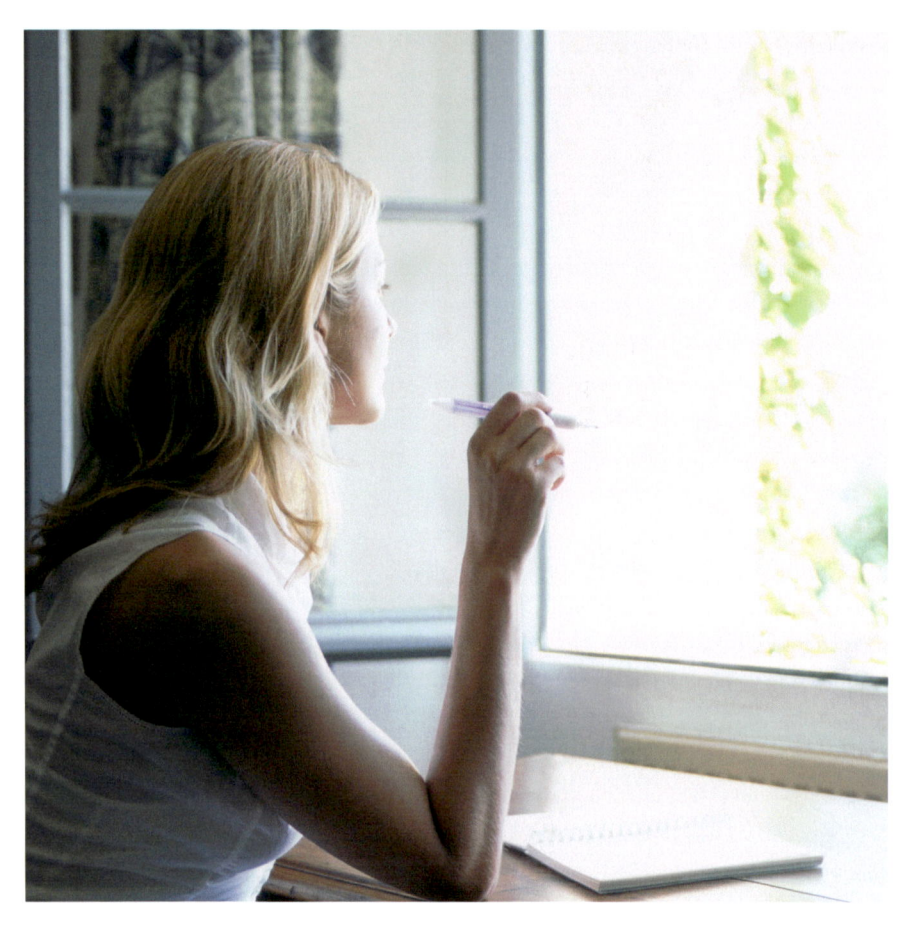

Use the colours in your mind map to try and unravel some of your deeper emotional mazes.

This stage, in which you try to identify the source of your feelings is at least half the battle. Go deeper than saying 'I'm angry because he didn't do the washing-up this morning.' Are you the one who always does the housework? Does this make you feel taken for granted on a fundamental level? It can sometimes be very tricky to put a finger on why we feel the way we do about someone, because toxic emotions frequently come from situations in our past rather than deriving wholly from the present scenario.

Analysing your emotions

Let's say, for example, that you have a troubled relationship with your father. Maybe he pushed you too hard as a child, wanting you to be more successful at exams or at sport than you were able to achieve, and so you always felt that you were letting him down. You either felt angry about the pressure you were under or you took in the message on some level that you weren't quite good enough, or both. Loads of people carry emotional burdens like this into adulthood, where it affects not just their relationship with their parent, but also with their partner, children, boss and/or employees.

Those people who had this kind of critical father might tend to choose a critical partner, because subconsciously they are still trying to win that unwinnable battle for approval so that they can at last feel that they are 'good enough'. They might even find themselves pushing the same high standards onto their own children, so the pattern continues down through the generations. Variations on this scenario can be played out in the workplace and in friendships.

Those people who had an inadequate or absentee father might find themselves looking for someone to take care of them in relationships instead of learning the lesson that we all have to stand on our own two feet. Individuals who had a fragile, vulnerable mother might have learned to look after other people instead of tending to their own needs, so they tend to pick vulnerable partners. However, relationships that are born of neediness can very quickly become unbalanced and problematic for both partners.

> **must know**
>
> **Live longer**
> A team of psychologists at Yale University found that those who feel positive about ageing live on average seven-and-a-half years longer than those who do not. They found that the hearts and arteries of elderly people who were exposed to negative ageing stereotypes did not respond well to stress. Positive thinking seems to be a more important factor in longevity than low blood pressure, healthy weight, not smoking and taking exercise.

8 Emotional detoxing

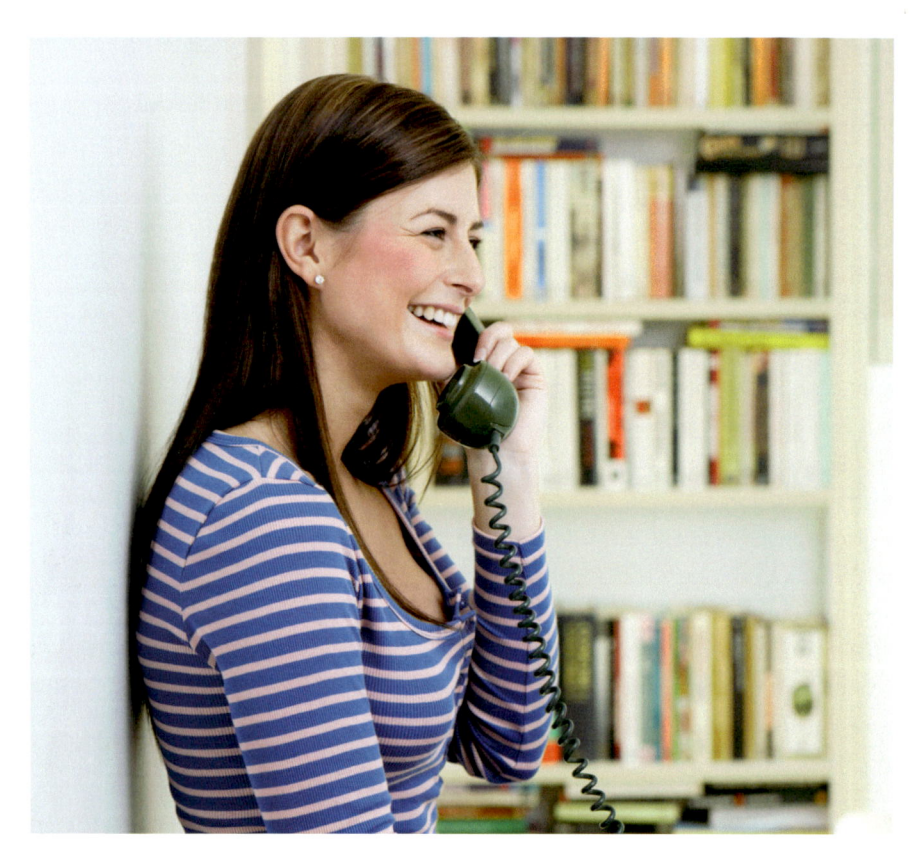

Respond to those around you as an adult, rather than trying to be a parent to other people, or acting like a child.

Childhood sibling rivalry can also extend into adulthood, when siblings become competitive over who has the bigger house or the smartest car, or whose children are doing best at school. If you learned to be competitive with a sibling in your childhood, you might find yourself creating similar relationship dynamics in adulthood, repeating the same behaviours and putting a strain on friendships as a result.

The kind of responses we learned in childhood, in order to survive whatever family dynamics were going on, can become ingrained eventually and spill over into our adult relationships, making them damaged and ultimately dysfunctional, because you are re-responding in ways that don't actually match the current situation. It can feel like being caught in a time warp. But what can you do about it?

Detoxifying relationships
The first thing to understand is that you cannot change other people. All you can do is to change yourself – but once you start behaving differently you might find that other people respond to you in a different way. To take one example: if your partner often belittles you, you can't directly force him or her to change. You need to consider ways in which you may be behaving like a child in the relationship and stop doing it. Start responding as an adult and it will be difficult for your partner to keep treating you like a child.

Modify your behaviour
Be aware that change is scary. Emotional detox can change your life. This is not the time to make huge changes like leaving your partner or selling your business, but you might start to modify the way in which you behave at work or at home, little by little, and consider the possibility of bigger changes over the long term. Here are some suggestions.
• Think about whether you are re-enacting childhood responses in your relationships and consciously stop doing it. Do the opposite. Cut through the emotion and react to the situation in hand. For example, if your over-critical father phones to tell you to update your car tax, do not immediately get defensive. Turn it on its head by

> **must know**
>
> **Me time**
> During a detox, start prioritizing yourself. Try to ring-fence some time to do things purely for your own pleasure. Maybe it could be going to a spa for a treatment or massage, or visiting an art exhibition or taking a bus to a part of town you have never visited before.

8 Emotional detoxing

> **must know**
>
> **Counselling**
> Some emotional issues are so painful and deep-rooted that you will need the help of a counsellor to untangle them. Opt for person-centred counselling to find a specialist who will look at you as an individual and help you to devise your own solutions. To find someone in your area, go to the website of the British Association of Counsellors and Psychotherapists (see page 187).

saying something like, 'Thank you for reminding me.' If your show-off brother calls to boast about his new car, congratulate him and ask if he'll take you for a spin some time. It's a powerful technique.

- Taking this a stage further: if you have trouble trusting in relationships, perhaps because someone cheated on you a long time ago, there comes a time when you have to consciously make a decision to change. Decide to trust someone if you really like them and don't give house room to doubts and negative thinking, which can be so destructive. You're a strong person; try to give your new partner the benefit of the doubt, instead of making them suffer for the faults of an ex.
- If a partner behaves badly, it may be appropriate to use the kind of behaviour modification techniques you use with small children: ignore bad behaviour – just walk away – and reward good behaviour with smiles, hugs and attention.
- Learn to say 'no' to requests that are unfair. Ask yourself, 'Would this person do this for me?' or 'How much gain is there for the other person compared to the loss or stress it would cause me?' When you say no, do so clearly, explain your reasons if necessary and don't go back on it.
- Sometimes it may be appropriate to weigh up a relationship in pounds, shillings and pence. Is the value all one way? Is it costing you far more than you are gaining from it? Would you be better off without it?
- If one particular resentment is poisoning a relationship, it's almost always a good idea to bring it out into the open. Try to frame criticism within a positive statement. For example, you might say to

a tight-fisted friend: 'I truly value our friendship and I love your company, but I've been noticing that I always spend more on our nights out than you do, and this has been spoiling my enjoyment. Maybe we could put the same amount into a kitty at the beginning of the evening so that we can relax and have fun without counting the pennies.' If they can't deal with your criticism, maybe the friendship won't be strong enough to survive but you will feel better for sticking up for yourself.

- If you are jealous of someone, why not tell them? Opening up in this way takes the poison out of the emotion, and they may confess in return that they are jealous of something you have.
- Set boundaries very clearly and stake out your territory. Let people know what you consider acceptable and what you don't as you go along.

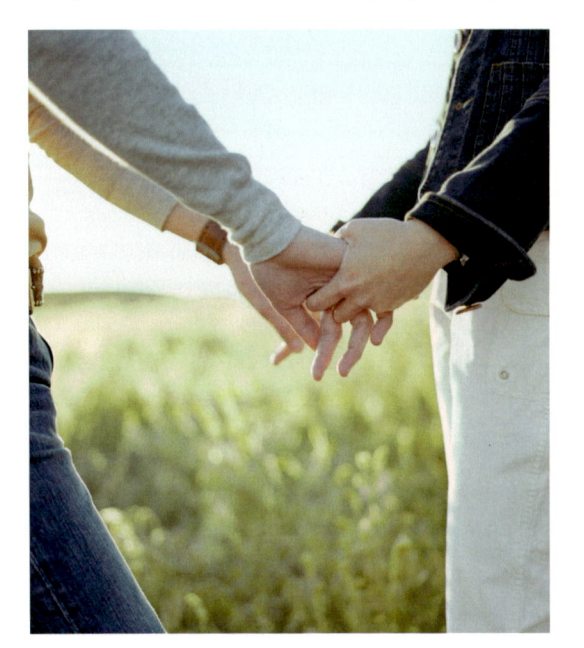

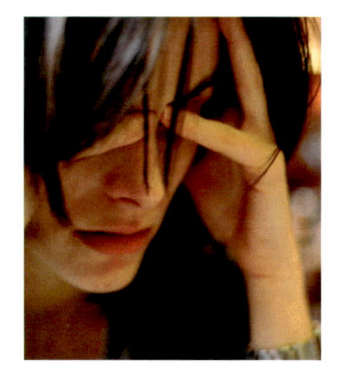

Don't brood endlessly. If someone has done something to upset you, confronting them can stop the resentment poisoning you.

Always meet others as an equal. Remember the Eleanor Roosevelt quote: 'No-one can make you feel inferior without your consent.'

8 Emotional detoxing

> **must know**
>
> **Write a journal**
> Some people find that recording the successes and frustrations of the day in a diary or journal is a very good way of releasing poisonous emotions. As you reflect on how to express what happened to you, you are already starting to rationalize and put it behind you. No wonder so many politicians keep diaries!

They will respect you far more for it than if you let them treat you like a doormat then explode with resentment from time to time over something minor that, for you, is the last straw.

- Learn how to negotiate in relationships. As in business, listen closely to what the other person really wants (which may not be what they are saying they want). Once you understand their needs, decide whether you are willing to accommodate them.
- You may decide you need some time away from a person with whom you have a toxic relationship. Stepping back to reflect can help resolve issues so that you go back stronger and more refreshed, ready to respond differently and deal with the situation more effectively. But when you go back, you are the person who will have to make the change.

Clearing the decks

Getting rid of emotional habits can take practice, but it's a good idea to start while you're on a detox. It's a time when you have cleared the decks to focus on your own needs, and emotional contentment should be near the top of your list.

Some people become addicted to dysfunctional relationships and trying to detox from them can feel like a major loss. If so, be kind to yourself and try to nurture other sides of yourself, such as your creativity, to fill the void. Be aware that when the detox is over you will still be at risk, like an alcoholic returning to the pub for an orange juice. Awareness and acceptance of the problem are a giant step in the right direction, though. Maybe the colour schemes on your mind map will look a bit different if you try it again in a few months' time.

Detoxing stressful situations

Make no mistake – stress is a killer. Our bodies respond as they did back in the Stone Age when a wolf entered our cave. Signals from the brain trigger the release of stress hormones adrenaline, noradrenaline and cortisol, which speed up the heart and breathing rates. Blood is diverted from the organs and skin to the muscles of the trunk, arms and legs that we would need to run away. Kidney function slows down; the salivary glands dry up; the liver releases more sugar and fat to provide energy for the muscles; digestion slows or stops. All these changes and more can take place in an instant.

If the stressful situation persists, cortisol increases our blood-sugar levels to keep providing energy, and aldosterone helps to keep the blood pressure raised so the body can keep its blood circulating. However, our supply of stress hormones is finite. The body has to produce them from scratch from the food we eat, to replace ones that are used up. After long periods of continual stress we can simply run out, a state known as 'adrenal exhaustion' in which blood sugar drops resulting in extreme fatigue. The delicate balance between the brain and the immune system can be damaged, since cortisol helps to regulate it, and the result can be an immune system overreaction that harms healthy cells and tissues.

Neutralizing stress

You will recognize from this description of the physiological effects of stress that most of them are the direct opposite of what you are trying to achieve when you detox and could even undo all your good

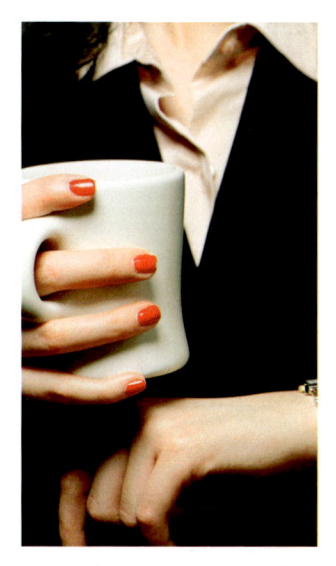

New technology, such as emails, texts and G3 phones, have made life move much faster so we frequently have to make instant decisions during the day.

> **must know**
>
> **Prayer**
> Some methods of prayer can be a form of meditation, when you empty your head of selfish thoughts and thereby open yourself to guidance from a higher power. If you are a religious person, you have a very powerful method of detoxing at your fingertips.

8 Emotional detoxing

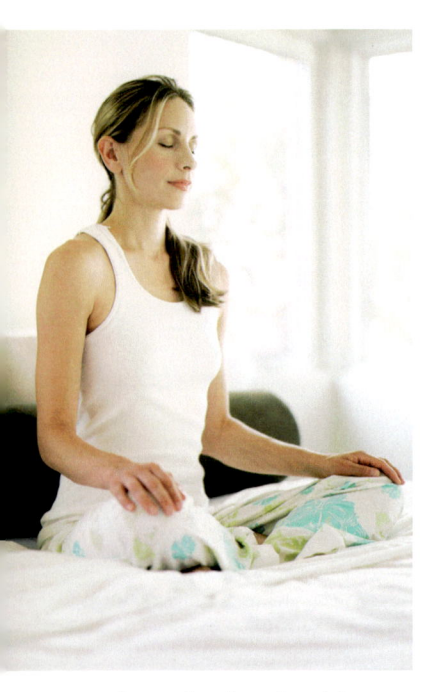

work. The solution is to seek ways of neutralizing stressful situations in your life and protect yourself if possible from such harmful physical reactions.

No one can be completely stress-free. We need a little stress to help us do our best in exams or driving tests, meet work deadlines and take on new challenges. So long as these stresses are spread out, with plenty of space between, the body has time to replenish itself. But if your daily routine has continual stressful situations, you need to change them.

How stressed are you?

- Do you commute to work through fume-laden traffic jams or stand like a sardine on a crowded train every morning? How can you change this?
- Do you have a boss who uses emotional blackmail or aggressive bullying techniques to pressurize the workforce? How can you change this?
- Do you live on a knife edge at home with an unreasonable, depressive or volatile partner? How can you change this?
- Are you over-committed in life, always rushing from pillar to post to keep up with all your responsibilities? How can you change this?

If you've answered 'yes' or 'I don't know' or 'I can't' to any of these questions then the truth is that you have to change your life or you could be killing yourself. Take a step back and start considering changing your job, working freelance or flexitime, starting your own business, getting more help with childcare, going to couples therapy, resigning from a few committees, shedding some responsibilities – whatever it takes to bring your life back to a more manageable level.

Researchers have found that physical changes take place in the body during meditation.

Stress-relief techniques

Having reduced obvious stressors, you must learn to deal with aggravating situations in a more 'chilled' way. There are several techniques that can help. Try the following exercises to see what works best for you.

Conscious breathing

Learning to breathe properly, with full inhalations and exhalations, has benefits for your whole body, including the heart, lungs, brain, circulation and muscles. Stand in front of a mirror and watch as you take a deep breath in. If your shoulders rise or your neck looks strained you are only breathing from the top of your lungs. Your ribs should expand outwards and backwards to accommodate the air, while your shoulders stay still. Try again, feeling the air pulled right down to your diaphragm and pushing your ribs outwards. When you exhale, they move back in again.

When you are in a stressful situation, stopping for a few minutes to focus on your breathing and thinking about where the breath is going can really lighten the load and counteract the harmful physiological effects of stress.

Close your eyes and breathe in through your nose right to your diaphragm. Let the muscles push the waste air back up again and out through your mouth. There are several useful breathing techniques you can learn, which are listed in the box (right).

Meditation

Devotees claim that 20 minutes spent meditating in the morning is the most valuable part of the day, the special 'me time' that gives them the strength to deal with whatever life throws at them. You can

> **must know**
>
> **Breathing techniques**
> • Astanga yoga uses a cleansing breath called ujjayi breathing.
> • Pilates and Alexander technique teach good posture and muscle control to support effective breathing.
> • Buteyko is designed to help people with respiratory problems, such as asthma.
> • Singing and drama lessons will teach diaphragmatic breathing to help you project your voice.
> • Or you could practise the assertiveness training technique of going to a field miles from anywhere and yelling at the top of your voice. It's said to be very empowering!

8 Emotional detoxing

use Buddhist beads and mantras if you choose, but meditation does not have to have religious connotations. You can just sit comfortably and clear your head. It's quite a tricky skill to learn, and you will definitely progress more quickly if you go to a class, but the basics can be picked up from a book or a tape (see page 190 for some suggestions).

While you are meditating, your pattern of brainwaves changes from busy beta-waves to slower alpha-waves, and there are a number of physical benefits that come with practice – blood pressure and cholesterol can be lowered and adrenaline levels drop.

One of the easiest ways to start is just to sit comfortably, following the regular rise and fall of your breathing and counting the inhalations and exhalations. If other thoughts drift into your mind, push them out and think solely of the breathing. This is known as a mindfulness meditation. The complementary one used by most Buddhist organizations is a loving kindness meditation in which you send out loving thoughts to the universe.

You can do a quick meditation session in the office whenever you need to clear your head, or on the packed train or bus ride home, or at night in bed when you can't get to sleep because your brain won't shut down, but most meditators claim that the morning session is the most beneficial.

More stress-relief suggestions

Here are a few more ideas that may help you to relieve the stress in your life.
- Exercise of any kind, whether you are rushing around after a ball or twisting yourself into complex

> **must know**
>
> **Sex and traffic**
> Stuck in a traffic jam? Turn on the radio and listen to some calming music, and why not do some pelvic floor exercises at the same time? Both men and women need to do these to keep the muscles strong down there so they don't become incontinent later in life. The added bonus is they improve your sex life.

yoga postures, will counteract the toxic effects of stress chemicals and produce feel-good serotonin.
- Laughter is always good medicine. Watch your favourite film or TV comedies, call a friend to share a good joke or ask a small child to explain where babies come from – whatever it takes.
- Express your creativity – through dance, painting, music, writing, carpentry, cooking a delicious meal, decorating your sitting room.
- Physical contact with other humans or animals is a good tactic: cuddle a baby, stroke a dog, hug a friend, have sex or a good snog with your partner.
- Choose someone with whom you can set the world to rights in a long, honest conversation, either by phone or over the kitchen table.

Don't worry, be happy

The Mayo Clinic in the US identified four common forms of negative 'self-talk' that pessimists indulge in. These are as follows:
- Filtering – magnifying the negative aspects of a situation and filtering out the positive
- Personalizing – automatically blaming yourself when things go wrong
- Catastrophizing – automatically expecting the worst
- Polarizing – seeing things as good or bad, with no middle ground.

They suggest that pessimists consciously listen to their mental chatter and turn round the negative messages. Instead of saying 'I've never done it before', you say 'It will be a good opportunity to learn'; instead of saying 'There's no way it will work', you say 'I can try to make it work'. This technique

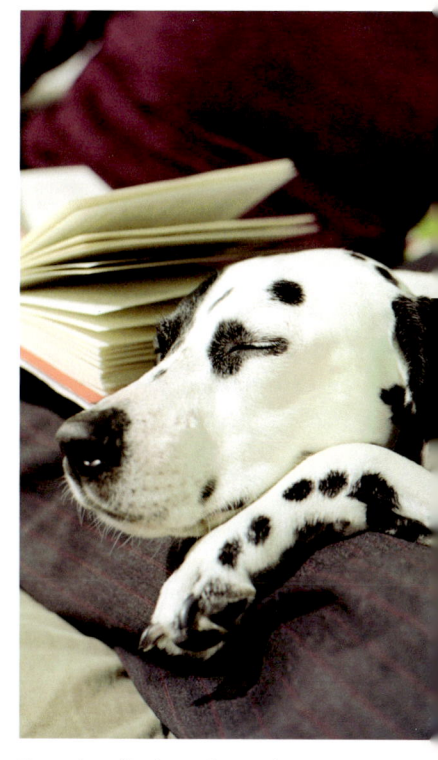

Several studies have shown that the simple act of stroking a dog can slow your heart rate and can cause your blood pressure to drop.

8 Emotional detoxing

> **must know**
>
> **Yes, but...**
> Eric Berne's book *Games People Play* identifies a number of different behaviour patterns to watch out for. One is the 'Yes but' game. Person A says that they have a problem and don't know what to do, so person B suggests 'Have you tried x?' Person A says 'Yes, but...' and explains why x wouldn't work. Person B says 'Have you tried y?' and person A again says 'Yes, but...' In fact, person A does not really want to change. Listen for this pattern in yourself.

requires self-awareness and lots of practice, but it is worth it if it succeeds in making you more optimistic because the benefits of optimism include decreased stress, improved health and longer life.

It may never happen

If we are honest with ourselves, a lot of stress in life comes from worrying about things that might never happen. What if... I miss the plane, or my partner gets ill and cannot work, or my children fail their exams, or my company goes bust, or I can't pay the mortgage and my house is repossessed. The list of things people worry about is endless – and worry creates stress, which makes us more toxic.

The next time you find yourself worrying about something that might never happen, ask yourself this: is the worry productive? By analysing the problem are you likely to come up with a solution that might help you to prevent the outcome you fear? If so, this can be valuable (but try not to lie awake at 3am doing this). However, there are a lot of stressors in life over which we have no control, and nothing we can do will prevent the feared outcome. When you find yourself indulging in this kind of worrying, *STOP*. Don't do it to yourself. Switch off and think about something else.

Overcome negative mental chatter

Easier said than done? A number of techniques can help. Deepak Chopra recommends a physical action such as clicking your fingers until the unwanted thought is sent on its way. You might come up with your own action, or choose a key word to remind yourself that you are indulging in 'negative mental

Opposite: Learn to enjoy the moment rather than brooding on the past or getting anxious about the future.

chatter' that will only cause you harm and will not solve anything. Why not abbreviate this phrase to 'Nemech'? Next time your partner is late home and you find yourself worrying that he/she has had an accident or is having an affair, say 'Nemech' firmly to yourself and move on.

Realize that every time you indulge in negative thinking, you are activating toxins that poison you physically as well as emotionally. The healthiest people in life are the ones who, in the words of the well-known prayer, 'accept the things they cannot change, yet have the courage to change the things they can, and the wisdom to know the difference.'

In fact, this prayer applies to the whole concept of detoxing, both physically and emotionally. We can't change everything and live in a perfect, purer-than-pure world, but learning what can be changed and taking steps to do it will make a huge difference.

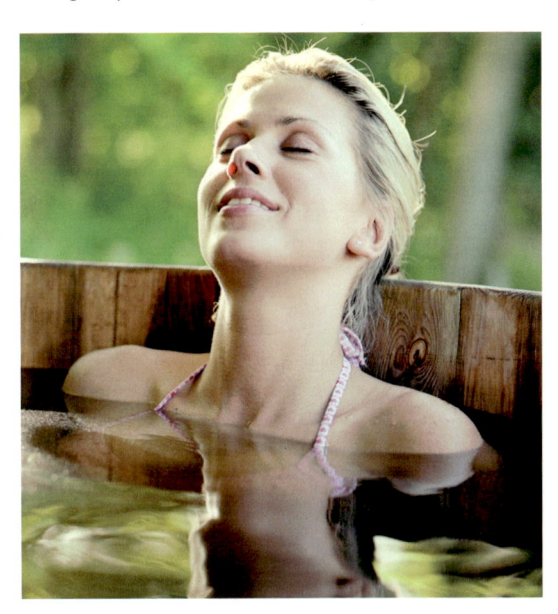

want to know more?

- Read Julia Cameron's book *The Artist's Way* in which she describes how to get back in touch with yourself.
- Read Daniel Graham's *Emotional Intelligence* to help develop your own.
- To find a meditation teacher, try The Vipassana Trust (01989 730234) at: www.dhamma.org
- The Transcendental Meditation Association: tel: 0870 5143733

weblinks

- British Association for Counselling and Psychotherapy: tel: 0870 443 5252 www.bacp.co.uk
- To find a counsellor, go to the website of the British Association of Counsellors and Psychotherapists: www.bacp.co.uk

Glossary

Acetaldehyde A toxic intermediary product which is created when alcohol is broken down by the liver.
Adrenaline Hormone released by adrenal gland in response to fear or stress.
Amino acids Building blocks of proteins, which we need to grow, repair cells and maintain muscles. Twelve essential amino acids are produced by the body, but we need to get a further eight from our food.
Antibody Substance produced by white blood cells to attack and neutralize invaders such as bacteria, viruses and other harmful micro-organisms.
Antioxidants Chemical that helps to neutralize free radicals and prevent damage they do to cells. Some occur naturally in the body; others are supplied by betacarotene, vitamin C, vitamin E and other nutrients.
Betacarotene Antioxidant that is converted in the intestine to retinol, which is essential for healthy skin and eyesight.
Carcinogen Substance that is capable of causing cancer, such as tobacco smoke.
Chelation Process in which chemical chelating agents are administered intravenously to combine with heavy metals in body and help neutralize them.
Cholesterol Fatty substance made by liver; used to form bile salts, hormones and other body cells; high levels in the blood can build up in arteries and cause them to narrow.
Cortisol Stress hormone produced by adrenal gland.
Diuretic Substance that increases the volume of urine passed.
Essential fatty acids (EFAs) Linoleic, linolenic and arachidonic acids are substances the body needs but doesn't produce (although it can make the other two from linoleic acid).
Food allergy Extreme immune system reaction to a food.
Food intolerance Adverse reaction to a food or ingredient in a food that can make you feel unwell.
Free radicals Unstable molecules with a negative electrical charge that cause cells to age and degenerate.
Glutathione Amino acid that enables the liver to break down several kinds of toxins, including acetaldehyde.
Healing crisis Syndrome in which symptoms get worse before they get better; during a detox this could occur when stored toxins are released into the bloodstream.
Heavy metals Metallic elements we ingest through food, air and water that build up in the body tissues.
Hypothyroidism Syndrome in which thyroid gland does not produce enough essential hormones, causing fatigue, intolerance of cold, muscle weakness, slower heart rate, and several other symptoms.
Immune system Collective name for the mechanisms by which the body fights invaders such as bacteria, viruses and toxic micro-organisms; also plays a role in the control of cancerous cells and is responsible for allergies.
Lactoferrin Antibacterial agent found in sweat, saliva and mucous membranes in the respiratory system.
Lymphatic system System of vessels in which lymph fluid is drained from body tissues and white blood cells are directed to areas where they are required to fight invaders.
Oestrogen dominance Syndrome found in men and women in which exposure to oestrogen in water and common foods leads to it becoming the dominant sex hormone.
Parabens Preservatives used in cosmetics and personal care products such as deodorants.
Phthalate Substance added to plastics to make them more flexible, and a solvent used in several cosmetic products.
Phytonutrients Nutrients that come from plants.
Placebo Chemically inert substance given to a control group during drug tests; it can have a positive effect simply because patient believes it will.
Probiotics Beneficial micro-organisms in digestive tract and help protect it from bacteria, yeasts and viruses.
Volatile organic compounds (VOCs) Substances used widely in paint, paint strippers, petrol, aerosol sprays, dry-cleaning fluid and many other common household products.

Need to know more?

Action on Smoking and Health (ASH)
102 Clifton Street,
London EC2A 4HW
Tel: 0800 169 0169
www.ash.org.uk

Alcoholics Anonymous
PO Box 1
Stonebow House, Stonebow,
York YO1 7NJ
Tel: 0845 769 7555
www.alcoholics-anonymous.org.uk

Allergy UK
3 White Oak Square,
London Road, Swanley,
Kent BR8 7AG
Helpline 01322 619898
www.allergyuk.org

Aromatherapy Consortium
PO Box 6522
Desborough, Kettering,
Northants NN14 2YX
Tel: 0870 7743477
www.aromatherapy-regulation.co.uk

Asthma UK
Summit House,
70 Wilson Street,
London EC2A 2DB
Tel: 020 7786 5000
www.asthma.org.uk

British Association for Counselling and Psychotherapy
BACP House,
35-37 Albert Street, Rugby,
Warwickshire CV21 2SG
Tel: 0870 443 5252
www.bacp.co.uk

British Heart Foundation
14 Fitzhardinge Street,
London W1H 6DH
Tel: 020 7935 0185
www.bhf.org.uk

British Nutrition Foundation
High Holborn House,
52-54 High Holborn,
London WC1V 6RQ
Tel: 020 7404 6504
www.nutrition.org.uk

Cancer Research UK
PO Box 123
Lincoln's Inn Fields,
London Wc2A 3PX
Tel: 020 7242 0200
www.cancerresearchuk.org

College of Naturopathic Medicine UK
Unit 1, Bulrushes Farm,
Coombe Hill Road,
East Grinstead,
West Sussex RH19 4LZ
Tel: 01342 410 505
www.naturopathy-uk.com

Friends of the Earth
26-28 Underwood Street,
London N1 7JQ
Tel: 020 7490 1555
www.foe.co.uk

General Osteopathic Council
176 Tower Bridge Road,
London SE1 3LU
Tel: 020 7357 6655
www.osteopathy.org.uk

Narcotics Anonymous
202 City Road,
London EC1V 2PH

Tel: 0845 3733366
www.ukna.org

National Institute of Medical Herbalists
Elm House,
54 Mary Arches Street,
Exeter EX4 3BA
Tel: 01392 426022
www.nimh.org.uk

Soil Association
Bristol House
40-56 Victoria Street,
Bristol, BS1 6BY
Tel: 0117 314 5000
www.soilassociation.org

The Transcendental Meditation Association
Beacon House, Willow Walk,
Skelmersdale, Lancs
Tel: 0870 5143733
www.t-m.org.uk

The Vipassana Trust
Vipassana Centre Dhamma,
Dipa, Harewood End
Herefordshire HR2 8JS
Tel: 01989 730234
www.dhamma.org

Useful websites

www.chem-tox.com
(research on the effects of chemicals and pesticides)
www.foodnews.org/tools.php
(information on pesticides used on fruit and vegetables)
www.dwi.gov.uk
(Drinking Water Inspectorate)
www.kombuchatea.co.uk
(for advice on water filters)

Need to know more?

www.andalucia.com/health/alternative-health
(descriptions of therapies)
www.thewellnessstore.co.uk
(for supplements, natural health and beauty)
www.highernature.co.uk
(supplements)
www.healthydirect.co.uk
(supplements)
www.nealsyardremedies.com
(natural health and beauty)
http://flowervr.com/
(flower remedies)
www.detoku.com
(foot patches)
www.natureswisdom.co.uk
(flower and light essences)
www.greenpeople.co.uk
(natural personal care products)
www.SoOrganic.co.uk
(organic shopping)
www.gogreen.cellande.co.uk
(a green directory)
www.spiritofnature.co.uk
(natural products, from clothes to cosmetics)
www.theremustbeabetterway.co.uk
(products for allergy sufferers)
www.botanicals.co.uk
(hair care)
www.honestycosmetics.co.uk
(as the name implies)
www.ecomerchant.co.uk
(sustainable building materials)
www.planetnatural.com
(organic gardening)
www.gaias-garden.co.uk/tips
(natural advice)
www.organicgardening.co.uk
www.ecopaints.co.uk
www.ieko.co.uk (natural paints)
www.earthbornpaints.co.uk
www.greenbuildingstore.co.uk

Further reading

General nutrition
Bodyfoods for Busy People, Clarke, Jane (Quadrille)
Encyclopedia of Vitamins, Minerals and Herbal Supplements, Brewer, Sarah (Robinson)
The Food Pharmacy, Carper, Jean (Pocket Books)
L is for Labels, Amanda (Hay House)
Not on the Label: What Really Goes into the Food on your Plate, Lawrence, Felicity (Penguin)
What are you Really Eating?, Ursell, Amanda (Hay House)
You are What You Eat, McKeith, Gillian (Michael Joseph)

Giving up bad habits
Allen Carr's Easy Way to Stop Smoking (Penguin)
Collins Gem Stop Smoking, Paul, Gill (HarperCollins)
The Easy Way to Control Alcohol (Arcturus Foulsham)
The Thinking Person's Guide to Sobriety, Pluymen, Bert (Griffin)

Detox guides
Carol Vorderman's Detox Recipes (Virgin)
Carol Vorderman's 30-day Cellulite Plan (Virgin)
Detox: How to Cleanse and Revitalise your Body, your Home and your Life (Rodale)
Detox for Life, Vorderman, Carol (Virgin)
Detox Yourself, Scrivner, Jane (Piatkus)
Dr Joshi's Holistic Detox (Hodder)
The Fast Track Detox Diet, Gittleman, Ann Louise (Century)
La Stone Therapy Manual, Scrivner, Jane (Piatkus)
The Liver Detox Plan, Williams, Xandria (Vermilion)
The New Raw Energy, Kenton, Leslie (Vermilion)
Power Juices, Kenton, Leslie (Vermilion)
Total Detox: 6 Ways to Revitalise Your Life, Scrivner, Jane (Piatkus)

Organic living
A Field Guide to Buying Organic, Perry, Luddene and Schultz, Dan (Bantam)
A Healthy House – Naturally, Sullivan, Karen
It's Easy Being Green, Trask, Crissy (Gibbs Smith)
Naturally Clean, Hollender, Jeffrey (New Society)
Organic Housekeeping, Sandbeck, Ellen (Scribner)
The Really Good Life, Soil Association (Cassell)
Toxic Childhood, Palmer, Sue (Orion)

Emotional health
After the Ecstasy, the Laundry, Kornfield, Jack (Bantam)
The Artist's Way, Cameron, Julia (Jeremy P. Tarcher)
Emotional Intelligence, Golman, Daniel P. (Bantam)
Games People Play, Berne, Eric (Penguin)
Guided Meditations for Calmness, Awareness and Love, Bodhipaksa (Wisdom Books)
Meditation for Beginners, Kornfield, Jack (Bantam)
The Seven Spiritual Laws of Success, Chopra, Deepak (Excel Books)
Teach Yourself to Meditate, Harrison, Eric (Piatkus)

Index

air pollution 40, 166–169
alcohol 21, 24, 25, 29, 34, 35, 36, 40, 45, 53, 55, 61, 62, 119, 121, 138
allergies 18, 20, 22, 140, 156
aloe vera 120, 121
aluminium 14, 156
Alzheimer's disease 14, 156, 157
antibiotics 21, 59
antioxidants 40, 55
aromatherapy oils 128
artichoke extract 119
ashwaganda 120
asthma 9, 18, 19, 20, 29, 169
auriculotherapy 138
autism 14, 16
ayurveda 139–140
bath salts 127–128
bathing 126–128
bowel movements 11
buchu 120
cadmium 14, 16
caffeine 21, 29, 34, 35, 39, 40, 45, 53, 55, 74
cancer 19, 26, 28, 34, 39, 40, 41, 42, 45, 55, 58, 121, 152, 153, 156
chelation 134–135
cellulite 28
chlorine 16
coeliac disease 22
coffee enemas 136
colonic irrigation 135–136
conscious breathing 183
cosmetics 155–157
craniotherapy 145

dairy foods 34, 45, 51, 53
dandelion 120, 131
deodorants 155
detox kits 131
diabetes 26, 45, 75
digestion 9–10, 21–23, 38, 43–44, 75, 120, 121
dry cleaning 153
echinacea 118
emotional detoxing 172–187
exercise 46, 122–125
eyes 9, 26, 40
fasting 53
fibre 43–44, 55
flower essences 39, 129–130
fluoride 16, 66
food additives 14, 18, 59
food combining 52
foot patches 130
free radicals 40
furnishings 162–163
gall bladder 10, 46, 74, 138
hair loss 13
hair products 155
healing crisis 46, 145
heart disease 26, 39, 40, 41, 42, 45, 75
herbal supplements 117–121
herbs 39, 117–121, 131
hormones 13, 16, 20, 24, 28, 29, 120, 140, 153
hot stone therapy 141
household cleaning products 16, 158–161
hydrotherapy 145
infertility 29, 138, 153

insecticides 13, 163–165
irritable bowel syndrome 44, 121, 138
juicing 70–73
kidneys 10–11, 26, 45, 62, 117, 120, 122, 130, 160
Kneipp Method 147
lactose intolerance 51
laxatives 120
lead 14, 16
liver 10, 19, 24–25, 26, 34, 38, 45, 46, 61–65, 74, 116, 117, 119, 121, 122, 130, 138, 153, 160
lymphatic system 11, 122, 130
magnesium 63
manual lymphatic drainage 141
meditation 183–184
menu plans 76–79
mercury 14, 15, 16
fillings 157–158
milk thistle 119, 131
mineral supplements 116
natural cleaning 161
naturopathy 141
obesity 26–28
organic foods 58–59
osteopathy 145
osteoporosis 16
panax ginseng 121
Parkinson's disease 14
periods 13, 162
pesticides 14, 34, 58, 140, 167
phthalates 19, 155
prescription drugs 35, 36–38, 121

protein 34, 51–52
recipes 82–113
reiki 144
respiratory system 9, 20–21, 169
rolfing 143
salt 34
saunas 149
schisandra 121
seaweed baths 128
seaweed wraps 148–149
selenium 116
shiatsu 143
skin 11–13, 28, 41, 46, 121, 138
brushing 45, 55, 126
smoking 8, 13, 20, 35, 36, 62, 121
solvents 13, 24, 74
steam baths 149
stools 23, 43
stress 20, 28, 120, 181–187
sugar 34, 48
Swedish massage 143
tea 74–75
thalassotherapy 147–148
thyroid 34
tongue diagnosis 30
toxins 8–31, 152–169
traditional Chinese medicine 30, 46, 137–138
vitamins 40–43, 59, 62
supplements 34, 116
VOCs 16, 161
water 46, 54, 66–67
weight 26–28
loss 48
wheat 34, 46, 53, 76

Index | 191

Collins need to know?

Look out for these recent titles in Collins' practical and accessible **need to know?** series.

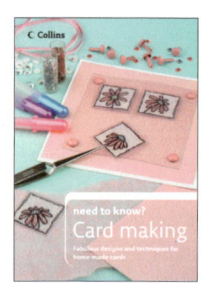

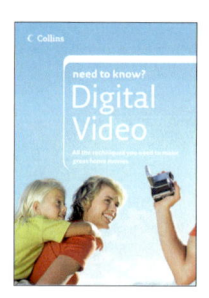

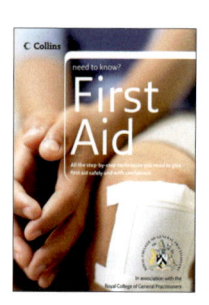

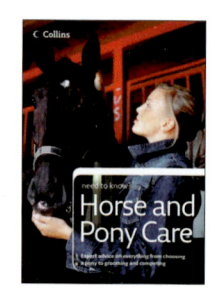

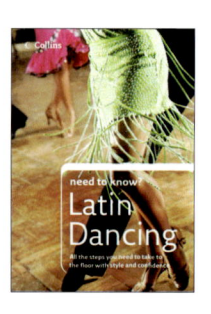

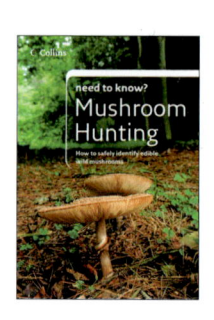

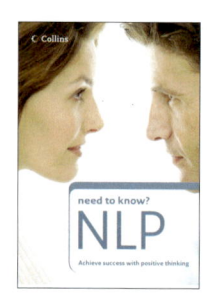

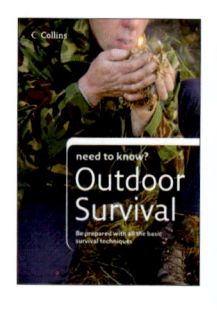

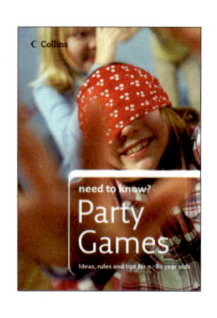

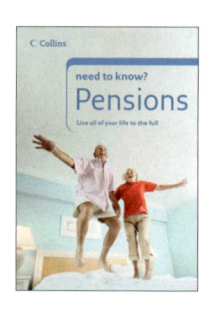

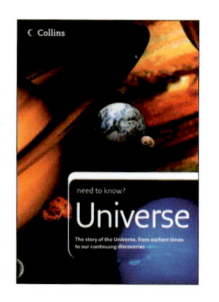

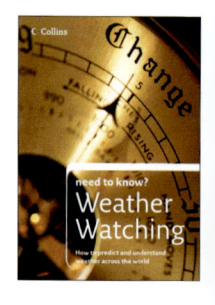

- Card making
- Digital Video
- First Aid
- Horse and Pony Care
- Latin Dancing
- Mushroom Hunting
- NLP
- Outdoor Survival
- Party Games
- Pensions
- Universe
- Weather Watching

Other titles in the series:

- Antique Marks
- Aquarium Fish
- Birdwatching
- Body Language
- Buying Property in France
- Buying Property in Spain
- Calorie Counting
- Card Games
- Chess
- Children's Parties
- Codes & Ciphers
- Decorating
- Detox
- Digital Photography
- DIY
- Dog Training
- Drawing & Sketching
- Dreams
- Food Allergies
- Golf
- Guitar
- How to Lose Weight
- Kama Sutra
- Kings and Queens
- Knots
- Low GI/GL Diet
- Pilates
- Poker
- Pregnancy
- Property
- Speak French
- Speak Italian
- Speak Spanish
- Stargazing
- Watercolour
- Weddings
- Wine
- Woodworking
- The World
- Yoga
- Zodiac Types

To order any of these titles, please telephone **0870 787 1732** quoting reference **263H**.
For further information about all Collins books, visit our website: **www.collins.co.uk**